BEYOND PAIN

Recent Titles in
Praeger Studies on Ethnic and National Identities in Politics

Using Force to Prevent Ethnic Violence: An Evaluation of Theory and Evidence
David Carment and Frank Harvey

The International Politics of Quebec Secession: State Making and State Breaking
in North America
David Carment, John F. Stack, Jr., and Frank Harvey, editors

Evolutionary Theory and Ethnic Conflict
Patrick James and David Goetze, editors

BEYOND PAIN

The Role of Pleasure and Culture in the Making of Foreign Affairs

THOMAS A. BRESLIN

PRAEGER STUDIES ON ETHNIC AND
NATIONAL IDENTITIES IN POLITICS
John F. Stack, Jr., Series Adviser

PRAEGER

Westport, Connecticut
London

Library of Congress Cataloging-in-Publication Data

Breslin, Thomas A.
    Beyond pain : the role of pleasure and culture in the making of foreign affairs /
Thomas A. Breslin.
        p.   cm.—(Praeger studies on ethnic and national identities in politics, ISSN
    1527–9901)
    Includes bibliographical references and index.
    ISBN 0–275–97430–8 (alk. paper)—ISBN 0–275–97431–6 (pbk. : alk. paper)
    1. International relations and culture. 2. Diplomacy. 3. Pleasure. 4. Pain.
I. Title. II. Series.
JZ1251.B74   2002
327.1'01—dc21   2001032904

British Library Cataloguing in Publication Data is available.

Library of Congress Catalog Card Number: 2001032904
ISBN: 0–275–97430–8
        0–275–97431–6 (pbk.)
ISSN: 1527–9901

First published in 2002

Praeger Publishers, 88 Post Road West, Westport, CT 06881
An imprint of Greenwood Publishing Group, Inc.
www.praeger.com

Printed in the United States of America

∞™

The paper used in this book complies with the
Permanent Paper Standard issued by the National
Information Standards Organization (Z39.48–1984).

P

To Agnes T. Oakes Breslin, source of my mother tongue; to the memory of my father, Joseph Patrick Breslin, who taught me my prayers in Irish and Latin; to Francis J. Dougherty, S.J., and Edward Murphy, who taught me Latin; to Francis X. Moan, S.J., who taught me Greek and Latin; to Edward Bodnar, S.J., and to the memory of Hayne Matin, S.J., who taught me Greek; to Daniel Brennan, who taught me French; to G. Ronald Murphy, S.J., and to the memory of Luther Brossman, who taught me German; to Gilbert Roy, who taught me Chinese; and to Gabriel M. Valdes, Frances Aid, and Maida I. Watson Espener, who taught me Spanish. Because of them I can say, as Homer wrote of Odysseus, that I "saw the cities of many peoples, and learned their manners."

Contents

Preface   ix

1. The Five Baits   1

2. Ten Thousand Persian Archers   21

3. Roman Virgins and Vandals   35

4. The Glittering Diplomacy of Byzantium   49

5. The Byzantine Doge and the Parsimonious Prince   67

6. Lording It over the Britons: England's Anglo-Norman Empire   85

7. The British Empire: Doomed in the Fleshpots of Paris   107

8. Whiskey versus Rum: The Roots of America's Bicultural
   Foreign Policy   133

9. Sweet and Sour: China Deals with the Modern West   163

Bibliography   179

Index   193

Preface

Humankind's history is bound up with pleasure. Pleasurable experiences can be strong enough to blunt the fears of deprivation and death that are the wellsprings of war. In an age when humankind has the weapons to destroy itself, histories that focus on pain to the exclusion of pleasure beggar the political imagination and narrow humankind's chances of survival. Under such circumstances, it is absolutely imperative to think beyond force and the principle of pain when considering government policy. Were pleasure in its culturally relevant setting acknowledged adequately as an effective diplomatic tool and often a cheap and safe one at that, then pain, which is ever more costly and deadly, might lose both its primacy and whatever shreds of legitimacy it may still have in this nuclear age.

This is a far-ranging historical study of the uses various cultures have made of pleasure in international relations. Pleasure, of course, manifests itself in various ways—sexual, psychological, celebratory, and gustatory, to name but a few of the guises in which we will meet it in such varied cultures as ancient and contemporary China, ancient and modern Europe, and contemporary America. The author makes no claim that pleasure is always stronger than pain in every culture, but to his knowledge the use of pleasure has almost never led to the downfall of a nation and the ruination of all its people. It is necessary to acknowledge that in the cases of some Amerindians and the Hawaiians their use of sex in diplomacy did expose them to venereal disease and contribute to their downfall under a barrage of deadly diseases against which they had no natural immunity.[1] In contrast, policies of pain have invariably crippled aggressor nations, immiserating all and sundry in the process and lately, as noted above, have even been threatening the annihilation of humanity in violation of the fundamental natural law that the human species must preserve itself.

Some novelists and lyricists of the twentieth century fearfully described how pleasure might be used to enslave. In theory, that may be true, but it is a path so different from that which humankind treads that such fear is a distraction from the far more threatening reality, a mosquito bite drawing the attention of a cancer victim. It is also more likely that a world in which policies of pain are foresworn for those of pleasure will be a world which has not only survived but has also met the hopeful challenge of the great Irish harper, Ruairi Dall O Cathain (d. 1653), in his song of reconciliation, "Is Tabhair Dom Do Lamh" ("Yes, Give Me Your Hand"), "people should be happy, joyful and free."

I acknowledge with gratitude the help of colleagues who have read all or part of the manuscript at one stage or another and made helpful suggestions for its improvement: Kathleen McCormack, Ramon Mendoza, William Marina, Maida Watson Espener, Nicholas Onuf, and John Stack. I also acknowledge with gratitude the help of the Florida International University librarians, particularly Ms. Marjorie A. Beary and Douglas F. Hasty. John Donohue coordinated the editing and proofing of the text.

NOTE

1. Alfred W. Crosby, *Germs, Seeds & Animals: Studies in Ecological History* (Armonk, N.Y.: M. E. Sharpe, 1994), pp. 120–147, esp. pp. 139–141, argues that the Hawaiians and Amerindians, who lacked Christians' and Jews' long experience with venereal disease, "used sexual favors as a currency in diplomacy and commerce just as they did and we do food and drink. (Indeed, we still use sexual favors to enhance negotiations, but not so openly as Hawaiians and Amerindians.)" As a result of this inexperience, these isolated peoples had "a lethally obsolete set of sexual mores" and were all the more exposed to the diseases carried by the Europeans.

1

The Five Baits

For millennia the Han Chinese struggled to dominate one another and their neighbors on the East Asian continent. Non-Han experienced their Han neighbors as flexible, martial, and relentless. Chinese military strategists developed an aggressive and effective military doctrine that stressed absolute flexibility in dealing with an enemy and had no compunctions about employing military force.[1] This martial culture continued to flourish as a sub-culture even after Confucianism, which favored accommodation in international relations and disdained the military, became the dominant culture of the Han. From 1100 B.C. to the fall of the last dynasty in 1911 A.D., the Chinese fought 3,790 recorded wars. The Ming dynasts alone during their 270-plus years in power (1368–1644) waged on average 1.12 wars per year against their non-Han neighbors.[2] Under their rule, the Han threw out the Mongols and once more were paramount in East Asia.

Alongside the well-studied military sub-culture was a diplomatic sub-culture that also played a notable role in Han expansion. It came to the fore in periods of Chinese military weakness. As flexible and opportunistic in its own way as the military sub-culture, the diplomatic sub-culture utilized pleasure in various forms as basic as sex or gold and as refined as the pleasures of the banquet hall to defend and even expand the Han living area. Sex, for example, was a powerful tool for the Chinese ruler. The foremost authority on the sexual practices of the ancient Chinese commented on the extensive use of sexual pleasure in their international relations. Robert Van Gulik reported that rulers kept "trained dancing girls and female musicians to entertain and engage in sexual relations with their master, his retinue, and his guests. They often changed hands, being sold and resold, or offered as presents. The sending of a bevy of beautiful dancing girls was part of the diplomatic routine among princely courts."[3]

Sexual pleasure was so effective in interstate relations that even Chinese military strategists included it in the study of their specialty. The thirty-first of one set of thirty-six military strategies used by the ancient Chinese was "The Beauty Trap." Kings often used exceptionally beautiful women to infatuate and distract the leaders of enemy states from the performance of their responsibilities. The smiles and tears of soft women would wear down rock-hard enemies. The author of another collection of military stratagems, "A Hundred War Maxims," included a chapter called simply, "Women." Of the usefulness of femininity this strategist wrote, "Employed in civil affairs, women can mislead and fool the enemy. Employed in military affairs, they can ride chariots to combat and relieve danger and difficulty. They are able to adapt to changing circumstances. Women move in where men are incompetent." In another work, "Six Strategies," a Chinese strategist widened the list of diplomatically useful pleasures: "The twelfth method is to cultivate the enemy's faithless courtiers to mislead him, offer beautiful women and lascivious music to infatuate him, present fine dogs and horses to fatigue him, submit flattering reports to blunt him, and seize a favorable opportunity and summon the people under Heaven to overcome him."[4]

Chinese women could be useful pawns in the Chinese diplomatic subculture, but they were also a threat. The notion that women could blunt the martial spirit of rulers was not far removed from the belief that foreign women could weaken or even bring down a Chinese ruling house. Chinese historians pointed to the fate of You, last ruler of the Western Zhou dynasty, as a warning against taking in foreign women and indulging them. When Zhou attacked the small vassal state of Bao for not providing tribute on schedule, Bao settled the dispute by providing ten beautiful women, the most dazzling of whom was the unsmiling Baosi. King You went to extraordinary expense to humor Baosi and even risked internal disaffection by making her his queen, but to no avail. Finally, at her suggestion, he lit a beacon fire, thereby summoning his alarmed vassals. Her pleasure at the anger of his abused vassals led him to light other beacon fires until the vassals no longer responded. In 771 B.C., when Western Zhou was attacked by northern enemies, its vassals refused to assist it. The dynasty fell, You was put to death, and Baosi was handed over to the victorious king.[5]

It would be difficult to exaggerate the role played by women in the relations of one Chinese state with another and in the relations of Chinese states with foreign states. Sometimes the role was one of temporary pleasure-giver, sometimes that of distraction, and more often that of long-term agent. During the tumultuous three centuries that followed the fall of Western Zhou, a time known as the Spring and Autumn period of Chinese history (770–453 B.C.), Chinese rulers tried desperately to build and maintain alliances that would maintain their small states. Armies alone were not enough. They brought their women into action. When the king of the relatively large state of Chu passed through Zheng in 638 B.C., the primary wives of the king of Zheng entertained him.[6] Zheng's position between the larger states of Jin and Chu left it exposed to frequent harassment. In self-defense it "used to amass large numbers of slaves and jade and silk objects at the border, and give them as state gifts to whomever came to cause a skirmish." The neighboring, weaker state of Song was less fortunate in its dealings with Chu. In the mid-sixth century B.C., Chu besieged it. Its subjects were reduced to swapping their children to eat as food. Prompted by a local anti-war movement in which two soldiers were prominent, Song persuaded Jin, Chu, Zheng, and other neighboring states to agree on a peace cemented by regular tribute to Jin and Chu.[7]

In that same period, the role of women in saving the state of Yue from eradication by the stronger state of Wu was more sustained and dramatic. Nearly defeated, with the Wu forces at his gates, the king of Yue was finally ready to listen to the advice of an official adviser and military trainer sent to him by his overlord, the king of Chu. At the adviser's suggestion, he bought the assistance of a favorite courtier of the Wu king with jade, gold, and eight beautiful women. The Wu courtier in turn persuaded his king to make peace with Yue. The Chu adviser, Wen Zhong, then laid out a seven-point strategy to undermine Wu and build up Yue. The strategy mixed sweet and sour: please Wu's king and ministers with money, demoralize the king with beautiful women, tempt him into wasting his resources on palaces by sending artisans, and confuse him with the flattery of treacherous sycophants. Meanwhile, buy grain from Wu's reserves to deplete them, sow dissent between the king and his capable ministers, and prepare for war. A hundred Yue courtiers secretly combed the country until they found a ravishing beauty to train in music, dance, court manners, and womanly arts. After three years of training, the woman, Xi Shi, traveled to the king of Wu as a gift of the king of Yue. The king of Wu became infatuated with her and neglected his duties. Wu entered into decline, and Yue ascended.[8]

There was, however, a more formal role for women in interstate politics. During this and subsequent periods of Chinese history, women often were the ties that kept alliances together. A woman given as a bride by one ruling house to another was, as Melvin P. Thatcher notes, "to use her influence to look after the interests of the state ruled by her natal lineage and in the long run to produce a line of heirs who would be amenable to maintaining friendly and supportive relations with it." To ensure that these ends were met, more and more states sent along with the young bride one of her nieces and one of her younger sisters to serve "as secondary wives and childbearers."[9]

The Chinese have never forgotten that women could use their sexuality to achieve dominance. A common Chinese expression for such a woman is "one who ruins city and state," a term first found in the Han dynasty in reference to Emperor Xiaowu's consort, Li. "In the north there is a beauty without peer. One glance from her could topple a city wall, another glance could topple a state."[10]

Important as sexual pleasure was in the history of China's international relations, access to luxury items and, above all, to food has been pivotal. Indeed, food and eating are central elements of Chinese culture. To overcome a climate of sparse and uneven rainfall, the Chinese instituted irrigation projects and borrowed agricultural technology from their neighbors. The resulting modest surpluses of grain and fiber, especially silk, attracted human parasites and traders from within and beyond China. Within, the reigning dynasty and its local followers usually carried off the surpluses, and often more. Nomadic neighbors from harsher areas sought to trade for grain, cloth, and iron or other metals. Denied trade, they would raid China and seize what they wanted from the peasants and artisans or those parasitizing them.

The accumulated production of humble Chinese villages made possible the military might and the elegant and awe-inspiring high culture of the various dynasties. While the quality of Chinese food has not been matched in history, the palace's food supply was bounteous and varied on a scale rarely matched in history until very recent times. The banquet tables of the emperor and, lately, of the premier were and are meant to create awe in a society tormented by local famines, where food has long been so much on everybody's mind that one customarily greets others by inquiring not merely whether they have eaten but whether they have eaten until stuffed. Imperial banquets were an unmistakable sign of overflowing power, the ability to command all. They impressed even those from countries where food was abundant.[11]

Every Chinese ruler from our time back to the Han dynasty and perhaps before that has grappled with the same dilemma: high culture with its awe-inspiring consumption seemed to depend on monopolizing the energy and production of the peasantry at the expense of the peasants themselves. Monopoly depended on warding off neighboring nomads and semi-nomads who might want to trade with the peasants or, denied that, steal from them. But tight trade restrictions against nomadic neighbors such as the Xiongnu and Mongols, or even skilled horsemen from mixed economies such as the Jurchen, led to war. War meant impressing peasants into military service and taking a great deal of land away from the remaining peasants to devote to horse breeding. Without the grain from that land, the empire had either to reduce its troop levels and its awe-inspiring consumption or to starve the peasantry until they revolted or became sick and died. Either result weakened the dynasty.[12]

Even if meant to protect the heartland, punitive military campaigns and especially military expansion of the frontiers were so expensive that they brought down one Chinese dynasty and government after another. Qin dynasty pursuit of the Xiongnu into the arid Ordos region of northwest China and exhaustive attempts to establish Chinese agriculture there led to peasant discontent that was the beginning of the downfall of the Qin. Under the succeeding Han dynasty, pursuit of the Xiongnu relieved population pressure but also exhausted the treasury. In the words of Owen Lattimore, the great modern historian of China's inner Asian frontier, "conquest and expansion were illusory. There was no kind of success that did not create its own reaction."[13]

For two millennia or more, Chinese strategists struggled with the problem and developed for the emperors various solutions to the dilemma. One approach was to reduce the cost of horses, an expensive military necessity, by buying them rather than by converting grainfields to pasture and breeding them. Another approach was to create military colonies that could grow their own food. Still another was to buy the support of some of China's neighbors and turn them against others. The Han dynasty did that with great success and expanded until it almost touched the Roman empire to the distant west.

The Han dynasty developed this approach only after some early misfortunes with more forceful policies. The first emperor of the early Han dynasty (206 B.C.–8 A.D.) launched a disastrous military campaign against the nomadic Xiongnu that nearly cost him his life. He had personally led an expedition against the Xiongnu and had beaten them in several battles. The Xiongnu encircled him and besieged him in the city of Baideng, in what is now Shanxi Province. The Grand Historian of the Han, Sima Qian, recounted that the Han emperor successfully bribed the wife of the Xiongnu leader to persuade her husband to end the siege and let the Han go away.[14]

Chastened, the Han emperor later took the advice of another assistant, Liu Jing, and in a settlement reached in 198 B.C. bought off his enemies. The Han promised to treat the Xiongnu state as an equal. The Chinese also agreed to make fixed annual payments of money, silk floss, fabrics, wine, rice, and other foods; they also promised a Han princess in marriage to the Xiongnu king. In return, the Xiongnu promised to stop their disruptive raids. For sixty years that policy, known as *heqin*, bought the Chinese imperfect relief.

The *heqin* policy was based on the premise that the Xiongnu were strong only as long as they maintained their nomadic, egalitarian ways and cavalry skills. Zhia I, a Chinese strategist, convinced his emperor that if the Xiongnu king settled down and adopted sedentary, class, and sex-distinctive ways, the other Xiongnu would imitate him, and Xiongnu society would grow corrupt, lose its military edge, and cease to be a threat to China. Indeed, the Xiongnu leaders would become dependent on the Chinese for the luxury goods whose ownership was a sign of power and authority, as it was in China. Except for iron, a crucial military item, Chinese luxury goods, like their courtesans, were especially unsuited to the life of the mounted warrior. Carriages needed roads; silk was ripped to shreds by shrubs that could barely scratch the nomads' customary leather and felt garb; grain was a bulky, heavy food, very difficult to store and to transport, while mares' milk and kumiss came from the very horses that gave the Xiongnu so much mobility; slaves, courtesans, and dependent females distracted and slowed down their masters.

Zhia I proposed what he called the five baits to corrupt the nomadic neighbors: elaborate clothes and carriages to corrupt their eyes; fine food to corrupt their mouths; music and effeminate women to corrupt their ears; lofty buildings, granaries, and slaves to corrupt their stomachs (i.e., slow them down); and royal banquets to corrupt their minds. Since broiled or roasted meat was so prized by the Chinese and their neighbors, Zhia even suggested that Han restaurants on the border include cooked meat on their menus to bring the Xiongnu, ancestors of the Huns who terrorized the West, over to the Chinese side. "When the Xiongnu have developed a craving for our cooked rice, keng stew, roasted meats, and wine," he wrote, "this will have become their fatal weakness."[15]

The Xiongnu understood that the goods and services of Han high culture were baits and that indulgence would cost them their ruggedness, and perhaps their culture. They indulged themselves anyway and grew soft and less willing to destroy the sources of the pleasures. For a while, they nibbled and nibbled at the five baits and eventually developed a huge appetite for them, so huge that they raided China for more. The Chinese policy thus occasionally backfired, but its long-term effects were just what the Chinese desired.

Rather than blaming the episodic breakdowns of the *heqin* policy on the great attractiveness of the baits or on other factors such as the treachery of their own generals, Chinese officials blamed them on the exiled Chinese eunuch, Yueh Zhongcang. When the emperor Wen (179–157 B.C.) dispatched a Chinese princess to the Xiongnu king, he sent Yueh along against his will. In revenge, Yueh tried mightily to warn the Xiongnu of the danger of the five baits. Failing to deter them, he was reduced to advising the Xiongnu on the quality of the Chinese offerings. His advice made it difficult to swindle the nomads and increased the cost of the program to China.

More expensive still than the five baits, but less readily acknowledged, was the military system backing up the *heqin* policy. Military costs were higher than they might have been and the military outlays sometimes made in vain, because some Han generals were disloyal and willing to defect to the Xiongnu or to enlist them against the Han dynasty. Ever more expensive outlays of silk and courtesans could not calm turmoil fostered by such disloyal elements, who at times seemed closer to the rough and ready Xiongnu than to the Han. So from about 133 B.C., Han rulers decided to sidestep their own treacherous military shield and use diplomacy to manage the Xiongnu. The new Han strategy was to reach behind the Xiongnu and buy the help of their neighbors to the west.[16]

The Han dynasty's most effective diplomat was Zhang Qian, who after 138 B.C. roved the western frontier setting one nomadic and semi-nomadic group against another. Though he twice fell into the hands of the Xiongnu, he managed to divide them and lure them to ruin.

After 60 B.C., the divided and weakened Xiongnu fell out among themselves and eventually divided into northern and southern branches. Defeated by their cousins, the southerners sought the protection of the Han. In return for abandoning any pretense to an equal relationship and taking on a tributary role, the southern Xiongnu received rich rewards from the triumphant Han dynasts. Once having given hostages and provided tribute, the southern Xiongnu king received immense gifts of silk, gold, clothes and grain, especially when he appeared personally at court to render obeisance to the Han emperor. In fact, the Xiongnu kings were eager to pay homage to the Han emperor, since the Chinese were ever more generous in responding to recurrent demonstrations of submission. In 51 B.C., for example, the

Han rewarded the submissive Xiongnu with 34,000 measures of dried grain, the largest single amount of dried provisions ever recorded in Han history.[17]

The toils of a clever diplomat and imperial largesse aside, credit for the decline of the Xiongnu as a threat to China must also go to the beautiful royal concubine, Wang Zhaojun, a tragic figure in traditional Chinese accounts. When the Xiongnu leader sought a Chinese princess, Wang volunteered to leave the court at Chang'an. After a great ceremonial marriage banquet, she left for the grasslands in 33 B.C. She soon bore the Xiongnu king a son. When he left her a widow after two years, Wang Zhaojun married his adult son and bore the son two daughters. She is believed to have worked continually for peace between the Chinese and the Xiongnu. Her daughters and grandson visited the Han capital, and for a half century after her marriage there was no war between Han and Xiongnu. Both Chinese and Xiongnu revered her.[18]

A royal marriage was not always a strategic option for Chinese diplomats. In the period following the Han, China split into three kingdoms: Wei, Wu, and Shu. Northernmost Wei was the strongest, and Wu and Shu often found it opportune to ally against the northerners. But their alliance was brittle. The King of Wu became suspicious of the Shu champion, General Guan Yu, whose army had occupied the Jingzhou district, a strategic area of the Wu kingdom, and defeated seven Wei armies in succession. To contain Guan, the King of Wu offered him the opportunity to give his daughter in marriage to Wu's son. Guan spurned the opportunity. Wu then secretly allied with Wei and cast about for a way to trap Guan. From the diplomatic arsenal, Wu chose flattery as his weapon. On his orders, Wu officers wrote such obsequious letters to General Guan Yu that the Shu general concluded there was no threat from Wu and abandoned his stronghold at Jingzhou. Wu then secretly occupied Jingzhou. Cut off from adequate supplies, Guan soon suffered defeat and death, a victim of his own carefully manipulated pride. Flattery had overcome the sword, and Guan's imprudence became a lesson for all Chinese on how to snatch defeat from the jaws of victory.[19]

The Sui dynasty succeeded briefly in putting post–Han dynasty China back together. Its second leader, Yang Guang, Emperor Yangdi, earned a notorious place in Chinese history as an extravagant leader whose excesses doomed his dynasty. Had his excesses been merely ceremonial, he would have earned a place in world history as the host of the world's first permanent resident foreign diplomatic corps. At his capital, Luoyang, Yangdi set lavish standards for diplomatic entertainment that Europe would not match until the Congress of Vienna in 1815, if then. Early in his reign (606 A.D.), he entertained the Turkic ruler, Qimin Khan, at an art festival by the Pond of Accumulated Green in the Park of Fragrant Flowers. To impress upon the visitor that China enjoyed peace and prosperity, Yangdi summoned his empire's musicians and performing artists to perform for the Turk. The grand show featured the country's musicians and the best of its artists. In the opening dance, performers costumed as a whale spouting real water swam toward the audience, then suddenly transformed into a twenty-meter-long dragon. The show so impressed the Khan that he asked to change into Chinese clothes and become an imperial subject. Yangdi refused; he needed foreigners to impress.

Eventually, there were more than twenty foreign envoys permanently stationed in Luoyang. Yangdi grandly feted them all and presented each with gold, silver, silk, and satin. Tribal chieftains followed, and Yangdi received them with even more pomp in celebrations that usually lasted a month at a time. Dancers, musicians, and acrobats performed on stages set up along the main street; 18,000 musicians performed in an open air theater. Lanterns illuminated the whole capital at night while foreigners and officials enjoyed the artistic entertainment. The display of wealth attracted foreign businessmen. Yangdi sought to impress them all the more by ordering the shops in Luoyang rebuilt or redecorated to an opulent standard. He had the trees along the streets draped in silk and satin to give the appearance of an eternal spring. He went further by ordering that foreign businessmen should be served only the best Chinese cuisine, free of charge, and be told that China was so wealthy that it was an earthly paradise where no one ever paid for food. The official explanation was as threadbare as the clothes worn by the readily evident poor folks. For, in the words of Luan Baoqun, "As Emperor Yangdi gloried in the successful display of the might of his empire, the ordinary people were squeezed dry by the government."[20]

The Emperor Yangdi's diplomacy was burdensome to the people, but his war making was far more so. He led his dynasty into the trap of fruitless military expansionism, and it quickly gave way to the Tang in 618 A.D. The shrewd, tough founder of the Ming dynasty (1683–1698 A.D.) pointed to the ancient distasteful lesson that military expansionism was a suicidal policy for any dynasty. Looking back from the perspective of more than a millennium, he wrote: "For example, the Sui [dynasty] Emperor Yang (600–618 A.D.) sent his forces to invade Liu-ch'iu [Ryuku Islands], killing and injuring the foreign people, setting fire to their palaces and homes, and taking several thousands of their men and women as prisoners. Yet the land which he gained was not enough to furnish him with supplies and the people he enthralled could not be made to serve him. For vain glory he exhausted China."[21]

The Tang dynasty, which succeeded Sui, once more drew Eurasia into sustained contact with a reunified China. Once again, high culture was put in the service of the Chinese state. Extravagantly wasteful banquets served notice that the ordinary and exotic alike were at the command of the emperor and aristocracy of China. The emperor's table was sure to have the most prized teas, those from Sichuan and Zhejiang. Having the best tea was important, because there was such a rage then in China for tea drinking that even visiting Turks rushed to the tea market upon entering the Chinese capital. From the troubled southern frontiers came the orange and tangerine. The Tang dynasts served not only Chinese food products but foreign ones as well. From Central Asia came the famous "mare teat" variety of grape sent by the Turkish ruler of Turfan and the golden yellow Samarkand peaches grown in the imperial orchards at Chang'an. These were edible proofs that the Tang could command the best foods from beyond the Chinese world.[22]

The emperor himself did not join in the elaborate banquets prepared to ingratiate and impress foreign tributaries and ambassadors, however much tribute they brought. He was a prisoner of an ancient tradition that no emperor should eat, drink, or listen to music in the company of foreigners. Although that same conservatism encouraged the emperor to eat traditional, often plain, Chinese foods, novel and exotic foods, including foreign foods, were enjoyed in the palace anyway.[23]

In the expansive early years of the Tang dynasty, Western goods were all the rage, and even the less wealthy could enjoy Western goods and entertainment. Wealthy Tang played the Western game of polo into the wee hours of the morning by the light of torches and, along with the less wealthy, delighted over pretty Iranian waitresses in the taverns.[24]

Even at its most vigorous and confident stage, when the presence of foreigners was a sign of the prowess of the empire, the Tang could not completely control their neighbors. So Tang dynasts used a loose rein (ji mi) with them, often employing contractual rhetoric that invoked ideas of friendship, legitimate interests, agreed-on frontiers, and the behavior and duties of diplomats, what Wang Gungwu suggests might be the rudiments of modern diplomacy.[25] The Tang treaty with Tibet in 821–822 A.D. was based on diplomatic parity. Sino-Turkish relations often were those of equality, but the Chinese were not above showering luxuries on their Turkish neighbors and attacking them when their leadership was too enervated to resist.[26] When pressed by internal rebels, the Tang bought help from the Turks with a marriage alliance. When the Khitan (Liao) threatened, the Tang bought them off with sixteen prefectures in north China, near present-day Beijing.[27]

The Tang dynasty, like the Song dynasty that followed it, is yet another example of a dynasty ruined by decisions to expand an empire through military means. In 751 A.D., the rising state of Nanzhao on China's southwestern frontier (in present-day Yunnan Province) drove back the Tang frontier forces from the upland jungles of the Yungui Plateau, and far to the west a Tang army suffered defeat in Central Asia at the hands of an Arab army. Central Asia was Islamized, and Chinese influence there declined. The overextended Tang were able to check the Turks in the West by relying on diplomatic means, the tried and true policy of divide and conquer. They repeated the triumphs of Han's hero-diplomat Zhang Qian. But as time went on, the Tang, like the Han before them, found their own regional military commanders less and less reliable and more and more treacherous. Finally, dependent on foreign troops, Tang collapsed in 907 A.D. Diplomacy had bought the Tang 150 years before it died of the cancer of militarism.

As the late Tang struggled with its own military, it became less open to the outside world. By the early ninth century, exotic foreign goods and services became scarce and expensive. Chinese culture began to become stifling. Artists looked back with longing on the Western and Southern contacts that had challenged their ancestors to look at life with a fresh, creative eye and ear. Tales of the foreign wonders became more and more exotic and "furnished to the nostalgic imagination what could not be granted to the senses." As one literary critic has written of the late Tang, "We are no longer in the world of flesh and blood. We are in the Dreamland in which the soul glimmers like the flame of a candle. The landscape has been transformed into an 'inscape.' The world is drowned in the immeasurable ocean of Darkness, and there remains only 'an odorous shade.' "[28]

The Chinese of the late Tang turned on resident foreigners, massacring foreign merchants.[29] This murderous distrust of foreigners went deep in some individuals. Even in earlier, more open times, one courtier of the second Tang emperor who favored a militarized approach to foreign affairs had written of the Xiongnu: "The Xiongnu with their human faces and animal hearts are not of our kind. When strong they are certain to rob and pillage; when weak, they come to submit. But their nature is such that they have no sense of gratitude or righteousness."[30] Meanness and cruelty on the frontier inevitably left their mark on Chinese society.

The successor dynasty, the Song, was less expansive than the early Tang and much less open to the outside world. It too, however, sealed its own fate by undertaking military adventures. Song did regain southern borderlands by crushing the Nan Tang empire. But for forty years it was frustrated in attempts to regain the northern borderlands given to the Northern Han, a vassal state of the Khitans' Liao dynasty. Although other states in Vietnam, Central Asia, and Korea sent Song tribute missions and were treated as inferiors, toward the Liao the Song behaved as equals in receiving their ambassadors and exchanging gifts with them.[31]

The Song were not satisfied with the peace of equals along the northern border. The dynasty was revanchist to the core. Liao's attempts to extend the hand of friendship encouraged only an uneasy peace. For four years Emperor Song Taicong wore a mask of cordiality which he finally threw aside in 979 A.D. to attack the Liao's vassals, the Northern Han. His goal was to take back the old Chinese lands near modern Beijing. Song Taicong was confident of Song power. Had not the arrival of tribute missions from Korea, Vietnam, and Inner Asia confirmed that power? Emperor Song Taicong pressed north, taking a recently arrived Liao envoy along with him. His forces crushed the Liao vassals but then on the site of modern Beijing were routed by the Liao. Song Taicong barely escaped. He marshalled his resources for several years and returned to the battlefield against the Liao in 986 A.D. He again suffered defeat.

After two resounding defeats at the hands of the Liao in seven years, Song Taicong took counsel of his advisers. Two advisers, Song Qi and Zhang Qi, presented him with differing analyses of the dynasty's diplomatic and military options. Song Qi advised trying to turn the Liao allies against Liao, the old divide and conquer strategy. While careful not to admit just how weak Song was, Zhang Qi counseled the emperor to imitate the Han and Tang when they were too weak to wage war and had to resort to diplomacy. They had put aside their weapons, spoken humbly, and sent generous gifts, including princesses, to obtain friendship and goods to establish firm bonds. This would buy time for the Song to build up a forward defense policy, but nothing more than that. Song Taicong and his son, Song Zhencong, followed Zhang Qi's advice halfheartedly, offering the Liao limited trading rights. The disgruntled Liao stayed on the attack for years and in 1004 A.D. launched a full-scale war that forced the Song to sue for peace the following year. The treaty of Shan-Yuan incorporated the terms of peace.

The ensuing peace between Song and Liao was based on annual Song payments of silk and silver, increased in 1042, and the cession of some additional northern land. The peace lasted almost 120 years, testimony to the efficacy of pleasure and accommodation that is all the more credible in light of the bankrupt policy of pain that Song had followed before 1005 A.D. The annual cost of pleasurably pacifying the Khitans was less than 1 or 2 percent of military expenditures in wartime.[32]

From ratification of the treaty the Chinese immediately moved to rectification of names, changing all place-names that suggested inferiority on the part of their northern neighbors or hostility toward them. They established a new diplomatic protocol recognizing the equality of the Khitans and carefully and systematically trained diplomats in the new practices. Both sides recognized a common border and negotiated disputes.[33]

Abrupt reversals of this order can induce a search for justification. Within months of the treaty, Chinese intellectuals began an eight-year study of the history of China's foreign relations that filled forty-five volumes of historical retrospective and analysis. Nineteen of thirty-four topics examined Chinese attitudes and policies toward non-Chinese. Song scholars looked carefully and found that China's rhetoric of supremacy was often misleading. When strong, China was arrogant; when weak, pliable in dealing with neighbors. Reflecting their culture's sense of superiority and the underlying strength of the martial sub-culture, the scholars themselves tended to be more comfortable analyzing situations where China was superior and found it impossible to renounce the rhetoric of superiority. They gave only one-sixth as much attention to marriage alliances, seeking good relations, treaty making, and trade as they did to war making and assertions of superiority. Nonetheless, the scholars urged a flexible, continuous diplomacy using the politics of pleasure when useful and resorting to war only to protect China's borders.[34]

When Song wavered from the path of peace to pressure the Xi Sha in 1042 A.D., it succeeded only in bringing down on itself overwhelming pressure from the Khitans to return to the treaty table and pay more for peace as noted above. From 100,000 units of silver and 200,000 units of silk per year, the price of peace with the Khitans increased to 200,000 units of silver and 300,000 units of silk per year. Since Song already enjoyed a large surplus in its trade with the Khitans, the increase in payments was easily borne. Indeed, Song lost not a unit of silver to the Khitans. The same general pattern prevailed in pacification payments made by the Song to the Xi Sha. By giving the rulers precious gifts, the Chinese created a market among all foreigners wishing to enjoy the same luxuries as their own rulers.[35]

In 1081 A.D., the Chinese court had Su Song, a former diplomat to the Khitans' Liao dynasty, compile a diplomatic history and handbook of Song-Liao relations. Su completed a very detailed and heavily documented work of 200 volumes two years later. Su pointed out with pride that peace with the Liao dynasty had "permitted the people in the border regions to live a normal life and reach old age without ever having been troubled by military actions."[36]

The meticulousness of Su, the diplomat-turned-historian, paralleled the care with which the Song put together and regulated their traveling embassies—all embassies were temporary at this time. They chose well educated, polished, healthy men as ambassadors. After bad experiences with riffraff chosen to accompany embassies as guards, the Song required that soldiers should not have a criminal record and should be good looking, as well as able-bodied and well trained; their officers should be in the prime of life, between thirty and fifty years of age.[37]

By local standards, Chinese emissaries were normally very well treated. In Korea, they were lodged in a guesthouse more sumptuous than the royal palace. The Chin lavished food on them and their entire retinues, feted them at banquets enlivened with music, dances, and theatrical performances, and received them with minutely detailed court rituals. They invited their guests to take part in shooting contests at which wine flowed freely. In Turkestan, Chinese diplomats could feast on the famous green-and-yellow-striped Persian melons of the Hami area, of which the Uzbeks proverbially said, "For procreation, a woman; for pleasure, a boy; but for divine ecstasy, a melon." And, of course, there was always and everywhere the customary official exchange of lavish gifts of precious metals, silks, embroidered garments, textiles, horses, jade, ivory, and, from the Chinese side, tea. No host would send off an embassy without lavishing gifts on the ambassadors and their escorts. Some hosts would provide the companionship of young females for ambassadors. On the negative side, Chinese envoys occasionally ended up prisoners in time of war, and in peace they were forced to endure local music melancholy to their ears and food not to their taste. The worst of the lesser indignities may have been participation in the drinking bouts customarily thrown by the Mongols for their honored guests, in the belief that drunken guests were of one heart with their hosts.[38]

The unwillingness of the Song rulers and their advisers to abide by this profitable arrangement with their northern neighbors led to a foolish attempt to use the Jurchen tribe against the Khitans. The plan backfired, and the Jurchen seized all of northern China, drove the Song south, and established a new dynasty, the Chin. The Chin forced the Song, now surviving behind the barriers of the Huai and Yangtze Rivers (thus earning the name of Southern Song in histories of China), to pay an annual tribute in return for peace. Once again, the Song managed to run a balance of payments surplus with a placated northern neighbor, because the Song tribute created an ever-greater market for Chinese goods. The Song had taken up the sword and badly damaged themselves again but had managed to buy survival with the profits of trade with Chin, with southern neighbors, and with overseas markets.

In 1206–1208 A.D., the Song again took up the sword in an attempt to take back China north of the Huai River. The campaign was a disaster and ended with payment of large Song reparations and the execution of the Chief Councilor to satisfy the victorious Chin. But by 1214 A.D. the Chin, as the Jurchen were called, were in trouble with their Chinese subjects and their neighbors. The Song tribute had intensified a love of luxury among the Jurchen. The Jurchen grew soft and fond enough of luxury to oppress their subjects and stir up discontent. Moreover, to pay for the luxury goods, they illegally sold horses to the Song, leaving too few in North China for the Chin government to mount adequate police forces and border guards. Banditry became common; the Khitans revolted, and so did the Chinese of Shandong; the Mongols invaded. Soon the Chin retreated to the old Song capital of Kaifeng.[39]

The desire for revenge so consumed Song courtiers that they would not hear of strengthening the Chin as a buffer state against the ever more powerful Mongols. Song cooperated in undermining the Chin and, finally, with 20,000 soldiers, took the field against the Chin while it sent the Mongols enough food to support their campaign against the doomed Chin. It was a terrible error compounded when Song made the fatal decision to wrest the barren north from the thinly spread Mongols. After decades of warfare against its erstwhile Mongol allies, Song, one of the longest-lived dynasties as a result of its pacification policies, passed from history in 1279 A.D., a victim of its own revanchism and resort to policies of pain.

The blood-drenched Mongol dynasty in turn passed into history at the hands of the Chinese Ming dynasty. The Ming, like all Chinese dynasties since the period of the Spring and Autumn and Warring States (ca. 800–200 B.C.), practiced a highly ritualized diplomacy that emphasized extravagant ceremonies of conspicuous consumption and gift giving.[40] The Ming employed more than a thousand cooks and assistants to prepare extravagant imperial banquets with dozens of courses and hundreds of dishes. All Chinese guests were seated in rank order according to their office or noble title. Envoys from states beyond the empire took seats ranked by the history of their nations' relationship to China. While the guests ate from the finest dining ware in splendid halls, they enjoyed spectacular performances by extraordinary dancers, singers, and martial artists. The banquets continued to have one purpose, demonstration of the emperor's command of the finest things under heaven.[41]

The Ming's pacification policy was not successful. Chinese terms for barter, whether or not under the guise of tributary gift exchanges, were not sufficiently generous to control the Mongols. In fact, some Chinese officials realized the problem and vainly appealed for more generous terms of trade rather than war. They lost the argument at the Chinese court. Subsequent military campaigns involving perhaps as many as 200,000 troops were not only very expensive but ineffective as well and cost Emperor Yonglo his life. The Ming then briefly resorted to generosity to hold their northwestern borders. The costs of a policy of trade, tribute, and intermarriage were at most only 30 percent of those of a militarized policy. Nonetheless, Chinese vacillation and tightfistedness led to still more warfare and military disasters, which on several occasions would have ended the Ming dynasty had not the Mongols fallen to fighting among themselves.[42]

In the northeast, the Ming were even more unlucky, and the same pattern of tightfistedness, vacillation, and pugnacity made enemies who did not tear themselves apart. Ming pacification worked well with the Jurchen, and the Chinese court greatly profited from the exchange until both sides began to pass inferior goods, local Chinese officials used force to extort personal gifts, and the Chinese government restricted the Jurchens' access to Chinese markets. Forty years of fighting ensued. Finally, the Ming resorted to generosity and bought fifty years of peace. But in 1541 A.D., desiring more profit from its relations with the Jurchen, who were well on the way to becoming the sophisticated and powerful people known later as Manchus, the Ming tightened its markets again and generated enough economic grievances to fuel an era of war.[43]

Vacillation between waging war and opening trade relations led to an expensive compromise—wall building. The walls became ever more lengthy and elaborate and were still being constructed when the dynasty fell in 1644. This attempt to isolate China from its northern neighbors served only to weaken China.

Reliance on arms and walls, the marks of its military sub-culture, instead of sharing the fruits of its high culture through gifts and trade meant that the Ming had to oppress the peasantry to pay for war.[44] The desperate peasantry rebelled. They were on the verge of taking over when a Chinese general, Wu Sangui, defected to the Manchus and invited them to enter China through the impregnable Shanhai Pass and crush the peasant rebels. The rebels had alienated Wu by killing his family and giving his ravishing concubine, Chen Yuanyuan, to their leading general.[45] The surprised Manchus, who had thrice failed to overrun China, started a long war that lasted for decades and devastated large areas of China. Eventually, the Manchus were victorious and established a dynasty that styled itself Qing, the pure.

NOTES

1. Alastair Iain Johnston, *Cultural Realism: Strategic Culture and Grand Strategy in Chinese History* (Princeton, N.J.: Princeton University Press, 1995), pp. 149–154.

2. Ibid., p. 27.

3. R. H. Van Gulik, *Sexual Life in Ancient China: A Preliminary Survey of Chinese Sex and Society from ca. 1500 B.C. Till 1644 A.D.* (Leiden, Netherlands: Brill, 1961; reprint, New York: Barnes & Noble Books, 1996), pp. 27–28.

4. Haichen Sun, comp. and trans., *The Wiles of War: 36 Military Strategies from Ancient China* (Beijing: Foreign Languages Press, 1991), pp. 284–295.

5. Tang Wei, "A Kingdom Lost for a Concubine's Smile," *China Reconstructs* 31:3 (March 1982), p. 72.

6. Melvin P. Thatcher, "Marriages of the Ruling Elite in the Spring and Autumn Period," in Rubie S. Watson and Patricia Buckley Ebrey, eds., *Marriage and Inequality in Chinese Society* (Berkeley: University of California Press, 1991), p. 29.

7. Hanzhang Tao, *Sun Tzu's Art of War: The Modern Chinese Interpretation*, trans. Yuan Shibing (New York: Sterling Publishing Co., 1987), pp. 74–75. Tao was a general in the People's Liberation Army and senior advisor at the Beijing Institute for International Strategic Studies.

8. Sun, *The Wiles of War*, pp. 284–295.

9. Thatcher, "Marriages of the Ruling Elite," p. 44.

10. Anne E. McLaren, trans. and ed., *The Chinese Femme Fatale: Stories from the Ming Period* (Sydney: Wild Peony, 1994), p. 1, citing Pan Gu, *Han Shu* (Beijing: Zhonghua Shudian, 1990; 12 vols.), juan 97A, 3951.

11. K. C. Chang, ed., *Food in Chinese Culture: Anthropological and Historical Perspectives* (New Haven, Conn.: Yale University Press, 1977), pp. 11, 15–16, 20–21, 50, 132–133, 157–158, 218, 280–287. Using the six criteria of culture, foods, dishes and methods, personnel, dining, and philosophy, cuisine scholar Lendel H.

Kotschevar rated Chinese cuisine first in the world, slightly ahead of French cuisine. See Lendel H. Kotschevar, "French and Chinese Cuisines: An Evaluation," *FIU Hospitality Review* 3:1 (Spring 1985), pp. 25–34.

12. For comments on the erroneous classification of the Jurchen as nomads, see Jing-shen Tao, *The Jurchen in Twelfth-Century China: A Study of Sinicization* (Seattle: University of Washington Press, 1976), p. 9.

13. Owen Lattimore, *Inner Asian Frontiers of China*, 2nd ed. (Irvington-on-Hudson, N.Y.: Capitol Publishing Co.; New York: American Geographical Society, 1951), pp. 497, 510.

14. Burton Watson, trans., *Records of the Grand Historian of China Translated from the Shih chi of Ssu-Ma Ch'ien, Vol. 2: The Age of Emperor Wu, 140 to Circa 100 B.C.* (New York: Columbia University Press, 1961), pp. 165–166. Apparently drawing on a more elaborate tradition, Congren Wang offers a somewhat different account. According to him, one of the Han emperor's chief advisers, Chen Ping, learned that the Xiongnu chief's wife was extremely jealous, so he "sent a picture of a beautiful girl to her with the message that the Han emperor would present the girl to the chief if the siege were not raised. Fearing that she would lose favor if the girl was taken into the chief's harem, she persuaded him to let [the Han emperor] escape." Congren Wang, comp., *Tales from the Imperial Palace of Ancient China, Vol. 3: Tales About Prime Ministers in Chinese History* (Hong Kong: Hai Feng Publishing Co., 1994), p. 92.

15. Ying-shih Yu, *Trade and Expansion in Han China: A Study in Sino-Barbarian Relations* (Berkeley: University of California Press, 1967), p. 66.

16. Ibid., pp. 9–11, 36–37; Lattimore, *Inner Asian Frontiers of China*, pp. 487–488, 36–39, 12–13; Yu, "Han China," in Chang, *Food in Chinese Culture*, p. 66.

17. Yu, "Han China," p. 77.

18. Tang Wei, "Wang Zhaojun: Was She Really So Sad?" *China Reconstructs* 32:7 (July 1983), pp. 65–66.

19. Tang Wei, "Guan Yu: The 'God of War' Who Failed," *China Reconstructs* 32:11 (November 1983), pp. 67–68.

20. Baoqun Luan, comp., *Tales from the Imperial Palace of Ancient China, Vol. 1: Tales About Chinese Emperors—Their Wild and Wise Ways* (Hong Kong: Hai Feng Publishing Co., 1994), pp. 297–300.

21. Morris Rossabi, *China and Inner Asia: From 1368 to the Present Day* (New York: Pica Press, 1975), p. 26.

22. Edward H. Schafer, "T'ang," in Chang, *Food in Chinese Culture*, pp. 94–96, 122–123.

23. Ibid., p. 133.

24. Edward H. Schafer, *The Golden Peaches of Samarkand: A Study in T'ang Exotics* (Berkeley: University of California Press, 1963), p. 21.

25. Gungwu Wang, "The Rhetoric of a Lesser Empire," in Morris Rossabi, ed., *China among Equals: The Middle Kingdom and Its Neighbors, 10th–14th Centuries* (Berkeley: University of California Press, 1983), p. 49. Note that Franke

finds the wellsprings of modern diplomacy at least a thousand years before. See Herbert Franke, "Sung Embassies: Some General Observations," in ibid., 139–141.

26. Ibid., p. 54; see also Jing-shen Tao, "Barbarians or Northerners: Northern Sung Images of the Khitans," in ibid., p. 67.

27. Wang, "The Rhetoric of a Lesser Empire," pp. 58–59.

28. Schafer, *The Golden Peaches of Samarkand*, p. 35.

29. Ibid., pp. 23, 28–35.

30. Wei Cheng (580–643 A.D.), one of Tang Tai Cong's closest advisers, quoted by Wang "The Rhetoric of a Lesser Empire," p. 49.

31. Rossabi, *China among Equals*, pp. 1–12.

32. Tao, "Barbarians or Northerners," p. 79.

33. Ibid., pp. 69–71.

34. Wang, "The Rhetoric of a Lesser Empire," pp. 54–63.

35. Yoshinobu Shiba, "Sung Foreign Trade: Its Scope and Organization," in Rossabi, *China among Equals*, pp. 99, 101.

36. Franke, "Sung Embassies: Some General Observations," p. 122.

37. Ibid., p. 123. Francois de Callieres, author of the early eighteenth-century French handbook on diplomacy, *On the Manner of Negotiating with Princes*, suggested similar criteria for choosing European diplomats. "It is also desirable," he wrote, "that an ambassador should be a man of birth and breeding, especially if he is employed in any of the principal courts of Europe, and it is by no means a negligible factor that he should have a noble presence and a handsome face, which undoubtedly are among the means which please mankind." Francois de Callieres, *On the Manner of Negotiating with Princes; on the Uses of Diplomacy; the Choice of Ministers and Envoys; and the Personal Qualities Necessary for Success Abroad*, trans. A. F. Whyte (Notre Dame, Ind.: University of Notre Dame Press, 1963), pp. 39–40 (orig. pub. Paris, 1716).

38. Franke, "Sung Embassies: Some General Observations," pp. 124–137. The Uzbek proverb comes from E. N. Anderson, *The Food of China* (New Haven, Conn. and London: Yale University Press, 1988), p. 223.

39. Tao, *The Jurchen in Twelfth-Century China*, pp. 84–117.

40. Franke, "Sung Embassies," p. 140.

41. Frederick W. Mote, "Yuan and Ming," in Chang, *Food in Chinese Culture*, p. 219.

42. Sechin Jagchid and Van Jay Symons, *Peace, War, and Trade along the Great Wall: Nomadic-Chinese Interaction through Two Millennia* (Bloomington: Indiana University Press, 1989), pp. 89–96, 108.

43. Rossabi, *China and Inner Asia*, pp. 39–59.

44. Arthur Waldron, *The Great Wall of China: From History to Myth* (Cambridge: Cambridge University Press, 1992 Canto ed.), traces the reliance on wall building to court politics. See especially pp. 171–193.

45. Sun, *The Wiles of War*, pp. 96–104.

2

Ten Thousand Persian Archers

Modern European civilization emerged after terrible struggles among a number of civilizations. The struggles lasted for decades or even centuries and sometimes led to the death of the contending civilizations. Narrow victories were not always enough to fend off exhaustion. The ancient Mycenaean empire became the prime example of this plight when it made a last desperate effort to capture Phrygian Troy and brought itself down in the process. From the blood and gore came Homer's epic *Iliad*, with its story of the Trojan Horse, and its sequel, the *Odyssey*, an epic ode to the triumph of guile and perseverance over sheer force of arms, and self-control over indulgence, in a world of wanton gods and cruel strangers separating the hero from his hearth and home.[1]

Homer's epic tales became the bedrock of Greek culture. Through them the young of Greece came to fear pleasure, particularly love, and to admire cunning and guile. Every Greek knew from the *Iliad*, the bedrock myth of Greek culture, that the catastrophic Trojan War came about because, when asked to choose the fairest of the goddesses, the shepherd Paris passed over the goddess of the austere virtue, wisdom, and chose the goddess of love, and a great war among mortals followed. A stratagem, the gift of the Trojan Horse, finally decided the epic war: The Trojans took pleasure in and celebrated an apparent victory by accepting a large statue of a horse as a gift from the seemingly defeated Greeks. They perished as a result. If this lesson were not enough, Homer followed it with the *Odyssey*, an epic about the adventurer Odysseus, whom the Greeks revered as their greatest cultural hero. The most pronounced characteristic of this survivor of the Trojan War was evasiveness, a description provided in the very first line of the *Odyssey*. Odysseus was "polytropos," an individual of many twists, a man who was able to twist his way out of almost anything.

As Homer told the story, Odysseus had ever to be on guard against the lures of the Lotus Eaters, the Sirens, and Circe. For him and his companions, the pleasures of opium, sex, and good food and drink were dangerous substances when offered by strangers. Some of his comrades died or were turned into swine because they were not as self-denying as he was. When he finally returned home, alone, he disguised himself and killed the suitors plaguing his wife as they reveled there in his, a stranger's, home. While they might take an oath to their own cities, the Greeks made this slippery, defeated soldier who learned he could not rely on his fellows their greatest cultural hero, and they made fear of pleasure a key concept of their culture.[2] But while strangers might use pleasure against them, pleasure in any quarter could be dangerous. As James Davidson puts it in his study of the consuming passions of classical Athens, the Greeks "saw themselves as exposed to all kinds of powerful forces. The world's delights were lying in wait to ambush them around the next corner. The pleasures of the table, eels and fried tuna-steaks, fragrant wine, and above all human beauty naturally exerted a strong influence on all those who came within their gravitational field."[3]

Fear of strangers, even and especially friendly strangers, and love of home made Greek culture self-conscious and hostile to outsiders. Even small differences among the Greeks led to strife. To lessen the strife and overcome the atomistic forces in their culture, the Greeks relied on hospitality freely extended as a courtesy by individuals to Greeks from other city-states to hold them together. Such private hospitality often flowered into individual friendships, *xenia*, and multiplied over time drew otherwise inward-looking city-states together into the reciprocal relationship of *proxenia*. This guest-friendship writ large became, along with ties of religion, loyalty, and sentiment binding mother cities and their colonies, the basis of Greek culture and diplomacy. The fundamental purpose of that diplomacy was the preservation of peace between the city-states. There were terrible exceptions, but Greek diplomacy was generally successful in keeping the peace among the city-states. It was less successful in building effective alliances.[4]

In the neighboring, and often threatening, Middle East, empire followed empire. The Greeks learned much from their neighbors and taught them a good deal, particularly the power of the bribe. Historians may marvel at the Greek hoplite infantry and fleets of triremes and pronounce them pivotal, but the Greeks' most feared weapon and their greatest weakness was the generous gift in the right quarter. When they forgot that aspect of their culture and especially when they resorted to arms to resolve their differences, they usually brought upon themselves tragedy.

The Greeks had openly displayed their cultural weaknesses to the Persians, who succeeded the Lydians as the political power dominating the eastern Greek cities. The Persians closely studied the Greeks. Knowing them to be divisive, venal, and superstitious, Persian rulers sought to take advantage of those weaknesses to divide and conquer the Greek city-states. When they exploited them fully, they defeated the Greeks; otherwise, they suffered terrible defeats.

Despite the Homeric warnings that were so much a part of their culture, the Greeks of the fourth century B.C. fell victim to the lure of Persian money, sometimes in the form of coins stamped with Persian archers. In the process, they sold out their fellow Greeks in Asia Minor. The important city-state of Miletus, for example, apparently at the instance of its priests of Apollo, who were probably bribed by the Persians, went over to the expanding empire. For fifty years thereafter, the Persian rulers seem to have bribed the priests of Apollo at Miletus and Delphi to make oracular pronouncements encouraging the Greeks to accommodate Persia. Furthermore, Greek city-states showed themselves willing to sell out imperial rebels who sought refuge in Greek cities. One by one, divided by jealousy and weakened by treacherous priests and by an equally treacherous merchant class lusting for the greater commercial opportunities of the far-flung Persian empire, the Greek states fell to a combination of Persian might, generosity, and guile.[5]

In dealing with the Greeks on their European frontier, the Persians soon fell into the trap of military expansion and set in motion the forces that led to the dissolution of their own empire. After putting down an uprising of Ionian Greek cities in Asia Minor, during which Greeks from Europe had attempted to help their Asian cousins, the Persian leadership determined that the Greek states ruled by tyrannies had opposed them, while those with democratic tendencies had been against war. The Persian leaders, therefore, encouraged the establishment of democracies in the Ionian cities and decided to eradicate the meddlesome anti-Persian tyrannies from Europe. They then advanced on European Greece, bribing priests and taking advantage of splits between tyrants and democrats to augment their military might. But the destruction of the temples of Eritrea, the mother city of Athens, and the enslavement of its people solidified the Athenians against the invaders. With little to lose, the desperate Athenians, aided only by the Plataeans, crushed the Persians on the Plain of Marathon in 490 B.C.[6]

The Persian leadership spent most of the next decade pacifying rebellious subjects closer to home and elaborating their magnificent capital. Then, under Xerxes, the Persians turned back to the task of conquering European Greece and expanding the northwestern frontier of the empire. Along with their armies and fleets, they deployed the customary bribes. The Apollonian priests at Delphi were on the Persian payroll and uttered effective pro-Persian oracles.

As the Persian invasion progressed in 480 B.C., half of the European Greeks submitted to the invaders by making ritual offerings of earth and water. The rest of the Greeks were divided. The Spartans feared that the Persians would infect their downtrodden slaves, the helots, with democratic ideas. They were determined to maintain their tyrannical way of life. But the Spartans could not convince the Athenians of their willingness to fight for anything but Sparta. A band of 300 Spartans and some allies confronted the Persians at Thermopylae. Learning that the Persians had stolen to their rear, the Spartans fought desperately to a certain death. "Tell them in Lakedaimon [Sparta], passer by, carrying out their orders, here we lie," read the stele later erected on the killing ground.[7]

Despite heavy losses from the desperate Spartans, the Persian army moved on against the divided Greeks and sacked Athens after overwhelming an Athenian rear guard. The Persian fleet was less fortunate. By forcing the divided and downcast Greek sailors to fight for their lives at Salamis instead of waiting for them to surrender as they would surely have done, the Persian king, Xerxes, lost a third of his 600 triremes, five times the losses of the Greeks. He then lost his composure and prompted much of his remaining fleet to desert by executing his captains.[8]

Xerxes left an army under Mardonius in continental Greece. When Mardonius acted, he committed once again the error of relying on military means to deal with the Greeks. Through lack of patience, he lost the opportunity to win them over by bribes and diplomatic efforts. Instead, once more, the Persians' military approach forced the Greeks into a desperate situation. Mardonius had half of the continental Greeks on his side. Making a show of military force, he destroyed Olynthus when it revolted against the Persians. Potidaea, in contrast, was too tough a nut to crack when it renounced its ties to Persia. Athens seemed even more formidable and its fleet a desirable addition to his forces, so he sent an old friend of Athens, Alexander of Macedon, to offer the Athenians complete forgiveness, money to rebuild their temples, as much additional territory as they desired, and equal alliance as a free city. The Athenian aristocracy was inclined to fight and called upon the Spartans for help. When the Spartans refused anything but relief supplies, the Athenian aristocrats were in a quandary. Under the circumstances, Mardonius' Theban allies advised him to bribe the Athenian leaders. Mardonius refused, plunged ahead, and the Persians captured Athens again. After the Athenians threatened to ally with Persia, the Spartans finally decided to fight. The news of the alliance enraged Mardonius, who had Athens burnt again and retired to Boeotia, where the desperate Athenians, Spartans, and their allies confronted him at Plataea in 479 B.C.

Advised to retire and use bribes to win over the thirsty, starving Greeks under the command of Pausanias the Spartan, Mardonius again refused. When they began to withdraw in disarray, Mardonius decided to launch a swift attack and annihilate the enemy. With the end of the war in sight, the enemy coalition apparently falling apart under his eyes, the Athenians sure to come to terms, and the rest of the hostile Greek cities easy prey had he held back, Mardonius sent his troops into what became a desperate battle.[9] Then Mardonius made the fatal mistake of personally entering the battle. His death broke the Persian army. A second Persian army that could have broken the weary, battered Greeks withdrew upon news of developments in Persia.

On the afternoon of the Greek victory at Plataea, the Greeks nearly annihilated a Persian force beached on the promontory of Mykale on the Asian mainland across from the island of Samos. The victory not only sparked a second revolt of some Ionian cities against Persia but swept the Aegean clear of Persian naval forces and established Athens as the leading Greek city-state in the war against the Persians. The defeat of a Persian expeditionary army on the far northwestern frontier at Plataea was crucial to the European Greeks but much less serious to the Persian empire than the loss of its remaining fleet and tributary cities.[10]

Consumed with desire to become king of all Greece, which he could only do with Persian help, the Spartan general Pausanias prepared to betray the Greeks. He sought in marriage a daughter of the Persian king whose dowry would provide the money for the bribes needed to achieve his dream. When his plan became obvious, the Athenians pushed the Spartans to indict him and also rallied the Greek city-states against Persia. Greek confidence that Persian opposition would be weak was well-founded on the knowledge that the pleasures and intrigues of the imperial harem were distracting Xerxes.[11]

The Spartans did try Pausanias but acquitted him of all the main counts, including collaboration with the Persians. Acquittal on that charge, according to Thucydides, flew in the face of very good evidence. Spartan willingness to continue in the war against Persia soon evaporated. The Spartans found the other Greeks no longer willing to accord them supreme military leadership, and they themselves feared that the Persians would corrupt other Spartan commanders as easily as they had Pausanias. Leadership in an anti-Persian war was an expensive, corrosive task best left to the Athenians as long as they were friendly. Pausanias pursued his Persian connection and brought ruin upon himself.[12]

In the years that followed, both the Persians and Greeks rebuilt their fleets and sought local advantage. Persia reestablished control over Cyprus, while the Athenian-led Greek allies cleared the Persians from Thrace. In 466 B.C., after a decade of hostilities and Greek political successes, a large Greek fleet under the leadership of the Athenian admiral, Cimon, sailed into Ionia. There they found the Persian Third Army weakened by reliance on Phoenician and Ionian Greek sailors, who remembered the fate of Persia's allies at Salamis long before. Deserted by the Phoenicians and betrayed by the Ionians, the Persian naval and land forces suffered annihilation at the mouth of the Eurymedon River. The tide turned against the Persian empire. Thus by 466 B.C., the Greeks, with Athens in the lead, took from the Persians all of Europe save one city and much of Asia Minor. Greek culture and influence spread rapidly through the latter region. Thucydides would point out to his fellow Greeks years later that the Persians had mostly themselves to blame for their failure to win continental Greece and hold Ionia.[13]

War booty poured into the Greek cities, alleviating their poverty. Athens in particular enjoyed the spoils of war. Its leaders beautified the city and its Academy, and strengthened its Acropolis. But as Davidson observes, "This very straightforward connection between wealth, pleasure and conquest meant that imperialism could be considered a rather dangerous game. Decadence was imported into the city along with all the valuable trophies, bringing seeds of decline with the harvest of war." In the next century Sparta would be corrupted by the "flattery and gold that accompanies imperial power." Xenophon would also note the same fate of Persia.[14]

Whatever pride the Greeks may have taken in their feats of arms, fear of bribery nonetheless infected their whole political life. Accusations of bribery became almost conventional. The great hero, Cimon, nearly fell victim to such accusations after he led an Athenian army to seize the mineral-rich island of Thasos in the northern Aegean. Athens was angered because Thasos was trying to secede from the Athenian-dominated Delian League of city-states. Athens also coveted the minerals, timber, and pitch

of the adjoining Thracian coast claimed by Thasos. When it went to war
for liberty and its claims, Thasos appealed to the Spartans. Distracted by
a helot uprising, the Spartans stayed out of the war, and Athens won. But
so greedy had the Athenians become that they impeached Cimon, their
victorious general, for not taking over neighboring Macedonia. His detrac-
tors claimed that he had been bribed into inaction. Cimon won acquittal.

Upon acquittal of bribery charges, Cimon successfully urged upon his
fellow Athenians a course of action that demonstrated just how carefully
Greeks looked over gifts from other Greeks. Cimon convinced the Athenians to dispatch him with an army to help the Spartans put down the helot
uprising. The Spartans, however, fearing that Athenian soldiers would
spread the democratic ideology in Sparta, sent word that they would solve
their own problems without help. Once again the slavery of the helots
proved the rotten core of Sparta. The rebuff was an embarrassment to
Cimon and sparked his banishment.[15]

Both Persia and its rival, Athens, soon were alienating their subjects with
heavy taxes. Egypt revolted against Persia and sought aid from Athens in
460 B.C. Eager to find a secure source of grain, Athens responded with
military support, even though it was spending heavily for land and sea
operations against Peloponnesian cities, including Corinth and Sparta, and
for massive long walls between Athens and its port, Piraeus. Persia countered by bribing the Spartans, who defeated Athens at Tanagra near Thebes
in 457 B.C. Athens turned to central Greece and crushed the Boeotian
League. Persia countered that with victories over the Athenians in Egypt
and the Athenian relief force in 454 B.C.

The overextended Athenian empire began to unravel. The Persians
sought unsuccessfully to win over the embittered Athenians with money.
An Athenian force under the rehabilitated Cimon fought a campaign to
take Cyprus. Cimon died in battle, and though the Athenians were ultimately victorious, both antagonists had begun to worry about the Spartans.
The Athenians under Pericles decided to make peace with Persia. The
"Peace of Callias," named for the head of the Athenian delegation to the
Persian capital, Susa, followed in 449 B.C. The peace was based on the
status quo ante bellum and established a demilitarized zone along the common border of the empire, limited the movement of navies, and embodied
an Athenian renunciation of future aid to rebels in Cyprus, Libya, or Egypt.
The treaty was a necessity for both sides but an embarrassment as well to
Athens. Callias was accordingly fined by his compatriots.[16]

Though the Peace of Callias proved short-lived, it encouraged an
exchange of knowledge that profoundly altered the consciousness of the

Western world. During its short span, Greeks, Persians, and Egyptians learned more about each other. Especially through the work of those intellectual giants, Democritus and Herodotus, African and Asian science and literature entered the Western canon. Asian and African religion also entered Greece at this time and had a powerful effect on Greek women.

By 445 B.C., Athens, under Pericles' leadership, was hard-pressed by revolt in Euboea and Megara and the threat of a Spartan-led coalition massed at the Athenian frontier. Pericles bribed the Spartan king and his adviser to lead the Spartan coalition home and to disband it. Plutarch, in his life of Pericles, notes that the Athenians accepted without question the mysterious expenditure of ten talents. He explained this sway over the Athenians by repeating Thucydides' explanation that Pericles' power grew out of "the confidence felt in his character, and superiority to all considerations of money." The Spartans smelled bribery in all of this. After studying the matter, they forced their king, Pleistoanax, into exile and pronounced a sentence of death on his adviser, Cleandridas. Cleandridas saved himself by flight. A generation later, his son, Gyllippus, was also accused of taking bribes.[17]

Having delivered Athens from the Spartan threat, Pericles then crushed the Euboeans. Subsequently, Athens made a thirty-year truce with the unreliable Spartans, giving over to Sparta nearly all of Athens' land possessions. Plutarch tells us that some historians believed that Pericles every year spent ten talents on bribes to the Spartan leaders to pacify them and to buy time for Athens so that it might be better prepared for war with Sparta. Pericles then began meddling in the affairs of Persia's north African colonies and Greek cities in the Persian empire. By 440 B.C., the Peace of Callias was in tatters, and Persia was resurgent in Asia Minor.[18]

In the sixth year of the Spartan-Athenian truce, according to Thucydides, war broke out between Samos and Miletus over Priene. The Milesians appealed to Athens. Athens intervened on the side of Samos. Plutarch believed that Pericles' deeply romantic feeling for his Milesian wife, Aspasia (who modeled herself on fellow Milesian Thargelia), was the reason Pericles led Athens into war against Samos. If so, love, the ever-feared *eros*, proved more powerful than money. For Pericles spurned a generous Persian bribe of 10,000 gold pieces to spare Samos. Instead, he undertook a perilous campaign that risked the Athenian empire to crush Samos.[19]

Notwithstanding the Persian threat, Athens and Sparta found it difficult to reconcile profound social and political differences. They grew increasingly estranged. Seeking information on developments at Athens, the Persian government sent Thargelia, a Milesian courtesan renowned for her beauty, charm, and wisdom, and some fellow courtesans to draw out the secrets of the Athenian leadership. With these same qualities, Thargelia had brought over to the Persian side the leaders of thirteen Ionian cities. The women were successful, and the Persian king relaxed and settled back to watch the Greeks tear themselves apart in the Peloponnesian War, which began in 431 B.C.[20]

Both Sparta and Athens sought Persian assistance during the ruinous, fratricidal war. Spartan diplomacy failed, because it was inconsistent.[21] The Athenians had more success and in 423 B.C. concluded a treaty of friendship with Darius II Ochus, King of Persia. The treaty had little effect other than perhaps to encourage the Spartans to end their war with the Athenians in 421 B.C. The ensuing peace was named after Nicias, the cautious Athenian general who advocated peace with Sparta.

Given the animosity between the leading Greek states, there was little danger that they would combine against the brittle Persian empire. Sure enough, rather than enjoy the peace, the Athenians recklessly launched an expedition against Syracuse that not only ended in disaster but brought the Spartans back into war against them in 413 B.C. Furthermore, the ensuing Athenian weakness tempted the financially strapped Persian empire to reclaim tribute-paying cities lost to Athens years before. Persia, however, first had to employ the traditional tools of bribes and soldiers to recapture some of its own Greek cities driven to revolt because of heavy taxation. Then it turned to perfidious Sparta for help in reclaiming Athenian tributaries.

Greed and ethnic pride struggled for control of Spartan foreign policy. The Spartans proceeded to break the Treaty of Miletus (412 B.C.), which they had signed with Persia, double-crossed the Persians, and kept all the tribute collected from Greek cities they had taken for Persia. The Persians sought to strike a bargain with the Spartans: a subsidy to underwrite the costs of the Spartan expedition in exchange for the captured Greek cities and their tribute. A second Treaty of Miletus embodying this transaction foundered, because the Spartans, in a rare fit of shame, were reluctant to give up the role of liberator for that of traitor. This reluctance could only have been strengthened when the Persians did not keep up the promised subsidy payments.

Persian generosity might have won the day, had it been employed. The Persians, however, decided to use quiet threats rather than inducements and opened negotiations with the Athenians in order to put pressure on the Spartans. The Spartans finally came to terms with the Persians: a temporary Persian subsidy and renunciation of claims to European and island Greece in exchange for temporary Spartan naval assistance and acceptance of Persian claims to all of Asiatic Greece. The bargain was struck.

Athens tried vainly to overcome the Spartan-Persian alliance. Against the advice of leading Persian diplomats, who saw clearly the treacherous nature of the Spartans, the Persian rulers put a large sum of money into Spartan military operations against Athens. Nonetheless, at first Athens gained victory after victory. But the Persians invested still more in Sparta, and by 405 B.C., the Spartans had cut Athens off from vital Russian grain supplies. By the next year, a starving Athens submitted.[22]

The triumph of Persia was short-lived. Persian dynastic instability, imperial overextension, and expensive meddling in Greek affairs set the stage for the decline of the troubled empire. Cyrus, a son of the recently deceased Darius, decided to seize the Persian throne. His grab for power was typical of the semi-barbarized frontier general who adds to his ranks the very barbarians he has been sent to control and then turns upon a central government distracted and threatened by other troubles. Such frontier-based traitors were familiar to Chinese dynasts and Roman emperors long ago as well as to heads of French, Spanish, and Portuguese governments in the twentieth century. To his own Persian troops Cyrus added 13,000 battle-hardened Greek mercenaries, jobless veterans of the Peloponnesian War under the command of Spartan General Clearchus. Thus strengthened, he attacked the central government as it was struggling to put down revolts in Iran and Egypt. Cyrus died in battle with King Artaxerxes. The Greek generals, save one traitor, were murdered by Artaxerxes, and the 10,000 surviving Greeks marched back through the empire to the sea as living examples of Persian weakness and thence into history as the heroes of Xenophon's *Anabasis*.

The Persian king now viewed Sparta as an enemy. Not surprisingly, when the Ionian Greek cities that had supported Cyrus appealed to the Spartans for protection from Persian retribution, the Spartans openly turned on their financial backers, assumed the mantle of "liberators," and went to war against Persia.

Clever diplomats using bribes, subventions, and lies played leading roles in the unfolding drama. Persia gave the Athenians money to build a fleet for use against Sparta. Persian diplomats induced the Boeotians not to support the Spartans and tricked the Spartan King, Agislaus, into a three-month truce by falsely promising peace with independence for the Greek cities in Asia. The Persians also bought the support of Thebes, Argos, and Corinth, three neighbors of Sparta in European Greece. Their decision, coupled with that of Athens, to go to war against Sparta forced Sparta to recall Agislaus to help defend the homeland. While the Spartans were on the defensive, a Persian-Athenian fleet installed democratic governments in Asian Greek cities lately under Spartan influence, and the Athenians rebuilt the walls of their city with Persian help. Yet when Sparta indicated that it would concede the Greek cities in Asia to Persia, Athens balked. Although Persia then gave Sparta money to build a fleet for use against Athens, there was soon war between donor and recipient. "Paid but not bought," conclude Adcock and Mosely of the Greeks so quick to take Persian money, likening the Greek statesmen to English politicians in the seventeenth century, who took "French money while they did what they thought best for their party or their country."[23] Bought or not, payment was effective as a short-term tool.

The Persian policy of pitting Greek against Greek led almost naturally to reconciliation with Sparta when Athens began backing rebels on Cyprus and in Egypt. Spartan and Syracusan fleets combined in 387 B.C. with Persian armies to wrest from Athens the Hellespont. Faced again with the loss of Russian grain and a recurrence of the famine that had ended the Peloponnesian War, Athens capitulated. The Athenians accepted a peace dictated by Persia that surrendered Cyprus, Clazomenae, and the Greek cities in Asia to Persia and made independent all other Greek cities except three islands once claimed by Athens, a gift meant to embarrass Athens. The Athenians agreed not to meddle in Cypriot affairs. The Peace of Antalcidas (386 B.C.), or the "King's Peace," as it was known, conceded to the Persian king the right to intervene in purely European affairs, a pitiful comedown for the Greeks and a victory for Persia that arms alone had not been able to achieve. It was the crowning achievement of the Persian empire on its northwest border and all the more remarkable as it came in the waning years of an empire afflicted by class warfare and outright rebellion.[24]

As for the Greeks, and particularly the Athenians, exhaustion of the soil, the toll of war and pestilence, and the spread of commercial competition left them with less and less but with careers in the military as mercenaries eager for booty to send home from Persia and Egypt, or wherever their services were in demand. The empires of Athens and Sparta passed into history.

While the wobbly Persian empire stumbled closer to the abyss, the Greeks had their revenge both culturally, as they would later have it on the Romans, and militarily. The Greeks had borrowed from the Asians and Africans, but they gave in return. Greek art, architecture, and dress, or lack of it, in the case of athletes, began to permeate western Asia and northern Africa. The Persian empire became more and more hellenized. Some of its

campaigns to suppress rebels were dependent on Greek mercenaries. Meanwhile, Athens formed alliances with disaffected elements of the Persian empire. Athenians and other Greeks helped the Egyptians free themselves from
Persian rule in a rebellion that lasted three years (385–383 B.C.). A subsequent campaign against two Cadusian (Iranian) rebel armies nearly cost
King Artaxerxes his life. Only the clever diplomacy of one of his generals
saved Artaxerxes and the Persian army.[25]

Fortunately for the Persians, the Greeks and the rebels alike could be
divided and pacified. The harshness of the Athenian empire toward its clients was notorious and counterproductive, driving some into revolt. But
the resurgent Persian empire was burdened with 115 sons of Artaxerxes'
360 concubines. The imperial succession of the ruthless Artaxerxes III
Ochus was notable for the slaughter of all of his relatives. With that blood
on his hands, he proceeded to crush the rebellious Cadusians. Following
that triumph, he demanded that his satraps disband their Greek mercenaries. This was enough to spur one of them, Artabazus, to ask Athens for
assistance in return for a generous gift. Though Demosthenes warned his
compatriots that the combination of Persian economic and diplomatic ability would once again split the Greek states, the Athenians took the money
from Artabazus and went to war.

After his troops were badly beaten on land, the Persian king cleverly
used other Greeks to rein in the Athenians. He ordered a fleet of 300 ships
to be assembled and made available to the enemies of Athens. The possibility of a sea war with other Greeks frightened Athens into peace. In
exchange for admitting the loss of her empire, Persia gave Athens two cities.
In the absence of an incorruptible leader like Pericles, money had once
again humbled force. The Persian King's "ten thousand archers," that is,
countless (myriad) coins with the figure of an archer stamped on them,
overmatched any number of well-armed and trained Greek heroes.

The rebellious satrap, Artabazus, next enlisted Thebes, once a supporter
of Persia. The Thebans were successful in the field, but Artabazus could
not conquer his fear that they would rekindle their pro-imperial sentiments
and subvert his troops, so he broke with the Thebans. It was a crucial
mistake. Soon he was forced to take refuge with Philip of Macedon (355–
336 B.C.), leaving Artxerxes III Ochus free to recapture Phoenecia and
Egypt. With the seas under Persian control once more, Cyprus submitted
to the empire.

Court intrigue and poison took the lives of Artaxerxes III Ochus and his
son, Arses, within a two-year span (338–336 B.C.). While Arses was still
alive, Philip of Macedon was assassinated, a deed of which some Persians

boasted. Philip had been planning a Greek crusade in Asia Minor. His son, Alexander, took up the cause but first had to reassert Macedonian power in Greece. The new Persian king, Darius III, lost a great opportunity to split the budding Macedonian empire when he turned down a request from Athens to finance a proposed revolt. Alexander then leveled rebellious Thebes to make an example of the fate in store for rebels. Darius finally tried bribes but could only buy Sparta and Demosthenes. Neither the Spartan phalanx nor the Athenian orator was able to turn the other Greeks against Philip. Darius, of course, did have some Greek mercenaries in his ranks.

Alexander invaded the empire of Persia with 35,000 troops. Initially, he butchered most captured Greek mercenaries and condemned others to slavery. As he advanced, the desperate defense of Greek mercenaries in Persian ranks convinced him to be more lenient as a way of winning over or lessening opposition. His conquest of Persia and its possessions was a close run thing and marked the end of an era. Persian diplomacy and Persian military tactics had failed to preserve the last of the great independent west Asian empires. The empire's great expanse had overstretched its core forces, and its voracious taxation had alienated too many subjects for it to survive. Its Macedonian successor, however, proved unable to overwhelm it by sheer savagery and had been forced by bloody experience to temper its attacks with inducements and mercy.[26]

As for European Greece, it never pulled itself together, even after the shrinkage of Macedonian power. Rather than resolve disputes among themselves in a peaceful fashion, the self-mutilated Greek city-states continued their old habit of appealing to an outside power to settle disputes, much like Central American nationals appealing to the United States two millennia later. Instead of invoking Persian help, they now invoked Roman help. Unlike the rich Persians who sent money, the much less wealthy, highly avaricious Romans sent troops to kill and steal.[27]

NOTES

1. A. T. Olmstead, *History of the Persian Empire* (Chicago: University of Chicago Press, 1948; 6th ed. 1970), p. 12. Except as noted, this chapter generally follows Olmstead's analysis of the Persian empire and its interaction with the Greek world.

2. John J. Winkler, *The Constraints of Desire* (New York: Routledge, 1990), esp. pp. 71–98, treats the fear of *eros*.

3. James N. Davidson, *Courtesans & Fishcakes: The Consuming Passions of Classical Athens* (New York: St. Martin's Press, 1998), pp. 142–143.

4. Frank Adcock and D. J. Mosely, *Diplomacy in Ancient Greece* (New York: St. Martin's Press, 1975), pp. 10–12.

5. Olmstead, *History of the Persian Empire*, pp. 43–44.

6. Ibid., pp. 158–161.

7. Andrew Robert Burn, *Persia and the Greeks: The Defence of the West, c. 546–478 B.C.* (London: Edward Arnold, 1962), pp. 421–422, provides a poetic translation of the anonymous couplet related by Herodotus.

8. Olmstead, *History of the Persian Empire*, pp. 250–255.

9. Burn, *Persia and the Greeks*, pp. 509–546, esp. pp. 525–527, however, makes less of distress within the Greek ranks than do Herodotus and Olmstead.

10. Here I adopt Olmstead's evaluation of the battle of Mykale being more important than that of Plataea rather than Burn's scornful rejection of that position. Burn's opinion of Olmstead's work springs from a narrow Hellenic perspective: "Olmstead, whose understanding of Greek history was clearly not on a par with his Persian, is very wide of the mark in speaking of a 'check at Salamis' but 'disaster at Mykale,' and in saying that 'Mykale and not Plataea was the decisive battle' " (*History of the Persian Empire*, pp. 253, 259). See Burn, *Persia and the Greeks*, p. 551.

11. Olmstead, *History of the Persian Empire*, pp. 262–271.

12. Thucydides, *History of the Peloponnesian War*, trans. Charles Foster Smith (Cambridge, Mass.: Harvard University Press; London: W. Heinemann, 1919), pp. 160–165, 214–229.

13. Olmstead, *History of the Persian Empire*, pp. 255–261.

14. Davidson, *Courtesans & Fishcakes*, pp. 280–281.

15. Adcock and Mosely, *Diplomacy in Ancient Greece*, pp. 30–31.

16. Olmstead, *History of the Persian Empire*, pp. 310–317; Burn, *Persia and the Greeks*, pp. 562–563.

17. Adcock and Mosely, *Diplomacy in Ancient Greece*, p. 37.

18. Olmstead, *History of the Persian Empire*, pp. 318–344.

19. Thucydides, *History of the Peloponnesian War*, 190–197; Plutarch, "Pericles," in *The Lives of the Noble Grecians and Romans*, trans. John Dryden, rev. Arthur Hugh Clough (New York: Modern Library, n.d.), pp. 200–204.

20. Olmstead, *History of the Persian Empire*, pp. 346–347.

21. Ibid., p. 354.

22. Ibid., pp. 355–371.

23. Adcock and Mosely, *Diplomacy in Ancient Greece*, p. 67.

24. Olmstead, *History of the Persian Empire*, pp. 371–397; Adcock and Mosely, *Diplomacy in Ancient Greece*, p. 70.

25. Olmstead, *History of the Persian Empire*, pp. 397–401.

26. Olmstead, *History of the Persian Empire*, pp. 486–496. Adcock and Mosely, *Diplomacy in Ancient Greece*, p. 97, see no reason to believe that Demosthenes was in Persia's pay.

27. Adcock and Mosely, *Diplomacy in Ancient Greece*, pp. 112–113.

3

Roman Virgins and Vandals

Roman imperialism took centuries to evolve. Its mechanisms went far beyond legions of brave fighting engineers. Not only brutality and rapacity but also shrewd calculation, persistence, and patient diplomacy characterized Roman expansion. So did pleasure and the fear of pleasure. Roman leaders studied their opponents and exploited cultural weaknesses. As the Persians had exploited Greek venality, so the Romans, for example, exploited Celtic venality. But the Romans did not limit themselves to the sword and the bribe. Roman victories extended wherever Roman merchants could create a taste for wine and other products of imperial high culture. Masters of organization, the Romans were able to undertake wars that lasted hundreds of years. As they expanded, however, they found that some of their softer tactics were turned back on them or had enemy counterparts. The Romans' successful two-century-long war against the Celts of Spain, for example, demonstrated the tenacity of the Romans and Iberians alike, as well as the ability of the whores, merchants, and soothsayers of the Iberian cities to demoralize the legionnaires. Only stern measures to distance the legionnaires from the purveyors of pleasure enabled the Romans to emerge victorious in Iberia.[1]

Roman expansion was opportunistic In fact, the Romans of the Republic and early monarchy preferred whenever they could to avoid fighting and to exploit divisions among their neighbors—*divide et impera*. To that end, the Romans were willing to buy the cooperation or at least the neutrality of their neighbors. Of course there were limits, and these at one point included a prohibition passed by the Roman senate in 230 B.C. against giving gold or silver to a Celt. The senators did not want the Celts to be able to upset carefully fostered balances of power by hiring mercenaries who might be used against Roman allies or the Romans themselves.[2]

Nonetheless, in emergencies the Romans could shower down gold on the Celts. In 171 B.C., the errant consul C. Cassius Longinus, in a mad quest for glory, led Roman troops from the northeastern Italian frontier across the Balkans to Macedonia, pillaging and enslaving along the way tribes allied to an important Celtic client, Cincibilis of Noricum. Loss of their support weakened Cincibilis and opened all of Italy to invasion. Disaster loomed. The Roman senate dispatched senior diplomats and lavish gifts of money, gold, silver, horses, and armor to Noricum. To further strengthen Roman ties to Cincibilis, they also bestowed on the Celts of Noricum the lucrative right to buy Italian horses and to resell them beyond the Alps. In doing this, the Romans ran the risk that hostile tribes might acquire the horses for raiding purposes. Diplomats of lesser rank hastened to the directly affected tribes to appease them as well.[3]

Whereas wanton behavior threatened the empire, individual and communal restrain could and did strengthen it. Thus accurate calculation of the costs and benefits of imperial expansion convinced the Romans to rely on diplomacy to keep open the passes through the unconquerable massif between Italy and the Rhone Valley. It also stayed Augustus from an invasion of Britain. Two centuries later, Dio Cassius complained that Septimius Severus had spent vast sums with little hope of return when he led an expansion into Mesopotamia.[4]

Distant riches were more attractive than barren lands close at hand and always tempted the Romans to abandon their careful international political calculations. Rome took control of Greece thirty years before finally clearing the Italian peninsula of organized opposition from Etruscans, Greeks, Celts, and other groups by defeating the Ligurians in 118–117 B.C. What the Romans found in the Greek heartland attracted and repelled them even more than what they had found in the Greek cities previously absorbed into the republican empire. Greece offered vastly more booty of all kinds, gold and silver, artistic works, and Greek slaves to amuse and educate the conquerors. Nonetheless, the Romans were uneasy about the fruits of their Greek conquests, and with good reason. The high and the mighty fought over Greek wealth, killing off many fellow Romans in the process. The surviving rich became richer, and the many poor became relatively poorer. Rich Romans used captive Greek teachers to educate themselves and their children. Soon the culture of Rome's upper classes become hellenized and ever more distinct from the culture of the Latin lower classes. Furthermore, these class divisions grew ever stronger, because Rome's legions and fleets soaked off so many resources that the lower classes and rural workers rarely could afford the education needed to participate in the relatively expensive Hellenistic culture.

Further accelerating the process of cultural disintegration, military expansion necessitated the recruitment of strangers and captured slaves whose values and beliefs were at great variance from traditional Roman mores. When prisoners of war and retired soldiers settled in Rome or other parts of Italy, their values and strange foreign religions with orgiastic practices early challenged Rome's martial values and its local religion, which was tightly laced with stoicism. As the number of aliens increased and they formed substantial communities within the empire, the staying power of their beliefs increased dramatically, and the cultural base of the empire eroded.[5]

Roman resistance to Greek and other foreign cultures was strong but very episodic. By 186 B.C., the Roman state began its efforts to curb foreign religions with a campaign to control the worship of Dionysus or Bacchus, the Greek god of pleasure. In 173 and 161 B.C., it banned the Epicureans from Rome, because they claimed that the gods had no interest in the affairs of men.[6] Moreover, the Epicureans espoused the beliefs that pleasure was the highest good, and that wise men avoided getting involved in public life. Such a creed threatened to turn good Romans into effete "greeklings," as Romans were want to disparagingly term Greeks.[7] Athenaeus tells us that, "The Romans, the most virtuous [manly] of men in all things, did a good job when they banished the Epicureans Alcaeus and Phileus from the city, in the consulship of Lucius Postumius [either in 173 or in 155 B.C.], because of the pleasures which they introduced."[8]

The Roman campaign against Greek and other foreign religions would continue intermittently for centuries. The worship of the eastern fertility goddess, Cybele, and that of the Egyptian goddess, Isis, especially challenged Roman values; so did worship of the charitable, suffering Jesus of Nazareth. The followers of Isis worshipped a female goddess and engaged in orgiastic religious rites. The loose behavior of the celebrants was a marked and subversive contrast to the discipline imposed by the empire on its soldiers and civilians. The Romans equated virility with self-discipline and femininity with lack of self-control. They believed that once females had experienced sexual intercourse they lost their *vir*ginity, their masculine self-control, and passed over to weak-willed femininity. The holiest group in Roman society was the group known as the Vestal Virgins. They had to maintain their virginity for a prescribed period of many years as an example of self-control for the whole society or suffer terrible punishment. Just as the Vestal Virgins exalted self-control and supported the discipline required by a militarized state, adherents of the feminist religions threatened the empire at its very foundation, the military. So did Christianity, because it embodied a message that condemned violence against neighbor and enemy alike. Furthermore, there was a widespread perception that the Christians' eucharistic feasts were no less orgiastic than those of the followers of Isis and Cybele. For a while Christian leaders went to great lengths to distinguish their religion from other foreign religions.[9]

Roman disdain for Greeks and things Greek ran deep, nourished by the Greeks' condition as beaten subjects of the Roman state. Like conquerors everywhere, the Romans found it practical and consoling to use ethnic stereotypes, generally negative, when talking about the subject peoples in their empire.[10] To them, the typical Greek displayed "[l]ack of good faith, lying, flattery, talkativeness and inept behavior."[11] In a Greek, Romans expected to find sloth, self-indulgence, and readiness to participate in drinking parties.[12] Greeks stereotypically were quick to use deference and flattery on their Roman overlords. If that did not succeed in softening Roman demands for financial tribute exacted by the much-hated tax collectors, Greeks were not above corrupting Roman governors with bribes of money and artworks.[13] Flattery, called by Cicero the handmaiden of vice and beneath the dignity of a freeman because it was used by men with an eye to pleasure and blind to truth, went to an extreme with the captive Greeks. They awarded the Roman emperor, Nero, first prize in the national competitions in music, athletics, and chariot driving. In return, Greece received limited freedom and tax-exemption.[14]

Of course, Nero was the emperor, but until the institution of the principate, the Greeks of Sicily and the eastern Mediterranean often had sought to soften their rulers and conquerors, Romans included, with the suggestion that they were semi-divine. Some Roman governors did not resist having their subjects dedicate games, or statues, or chariots to them. Others, however, such as Cicero in Cilicia, spurned such honors.[15]

Beyond flattery lay bribery, an offense against Roman law. Polybius observed of the Romans that although acquisitiveness was praiseworthy in their eyes, accepting bribes and showing greed for gain from unapproved activities were the most disgraceful things of all.[16] Yet Roman military forces were so rapacious that potential victims were more than willing to bribe their commanders and so escape being looted. Such peoples, particularly those of the relatively wealthy east, were ready with presents for the Roman conquerors, presents so expensive that they were easily recognizable by all as gross bribes. Those who took bribes laid themselves open to charges of theft and extortion.[17] In the west, the Germans were not above tempting the enemy. Julius Caesar carefully recounted that he spurned a bribe early in his campaign in Gaul against Ariovistus the German.[18]

While the Roman leaders counted on bribes and their legions to advance the boundaries of the empire and to line their own pockets, they were well aware that merchants and diplomats were very important agents in the maintenance and spread of the empire. Trade generated profits to underwrite the empire. Accordingly, Rome established the trading port colonies of Ostia, Antium, and Terracina. The ports' role in the nascent empire was clearly captured in the term given them, "*propugnacula imperii*" [the bulwarks of the empire].[19] Merchants served another purpose as well in Roman strategy. Like their Chinese counterparts, the Romans were quite conscious that their own trade goods rendered effeminate, softening up if not ensnaring, the neighbors of the empire. The success of the Roman and Italian traders and merchants who "served the needs and stimulated the tastes and appetites of rapidly Romanizing ruling groups of northern Italy" was but one early instance of many during the course of Roman expansion. It was not merely the personal enjoyment of the trade goods themselves that Romanizing elites enjoyed but also a degree of control, and profit, from the trade.[20] Again, the parallels with China and other empires are too clear to be overlooked.

Julius Caesar is our best example of a Roman militarist conscious of the enervating effects of trade on the empire's neighbors. He opened his *Gallic War* with the observation that the Belgae were the most courageous of the three nations of Gaul because they were farthest from the urbanized cultural areas along the Mediterranean coast and were least visited by Roman traders. The traders, he explained, offered for sale goods that would make them effeminate, literally, would render their [male] spirits effeminate. Caesar returned to the theme at the outset of Book IV of the *Gallic War* with the observation that the toughest of the Germans, the Suebi, heavily restricted trading and allowed no importation of wine because they believed that wine rendered men soft and effeminate, unfit for bearing hardship. Evidently, the power of Roman civilization over its neighbors was never far from Caesar's mind. In Book VI of the *Gallic War*, Caesar returned yet again to the theme of the emollient effect of civilization's pleasures on Rome's enemies. There he observed that the Gauls' proximity to Roman provinces and ready access to traders selling useful and luxurious items had softened them and set them up to be beaten in battle so often that they no longer thought of themselves as especially warlike.[21] Trying to summon the

Gauls to fight back, their leader, Vercengetorix, urged them to secure self-government and liberty by burning their buildings and destroying their grain hoards.[22]

Caesar managed to defeat Vercengetorix in the field, but despite many defeats the Gauls retained the capacity to rise up and take the field again. Against that possibility, Julius Caesar finally had to deploy the weapons of pleasure. He gathered together the Gallic chieftains, flattered them, paid them enormous bribes (*maximis praemiis*), and assured them that they would not be afflicted with additional taxes. In that way and only in that way was Caesar able to leave the area with his army and become a decisive player in Rome's internal politics.[23]

Caesar was not immune to the uses of pleasure in international relations, as Cleopatra demonstrated. By seducing Julius Caesar, Cleopatra, last of the Ptolemies, managed to have herself proclaimed sovereign of Egypt, as her father had willed, and to preserve Egypt's status as a client state of Rome. She bore Caesar a son, Caesarion, and he honored her at Rome. After Caesar's death, she bore Mark Antony three children. He favored her with additional land for her state. As the power struggle between Octavion and Mark Antony for control of the Roman world developed, Cleopatra became a lightning rod for Roman fears of foreigners, and especially the sensuous east. Her relationship with Antony became the pretext for a Roman declaration of war against her as Antony's enemies fomented fears that Antony would make her queen of Rome and remove the seat of government to Egypt, the ultimate steps in Oriental tyranny. Even with financial and military support from the east, Antony lost. Then, her rich offerings of money and sexual advances both spurned by Octavian, Cleopatra committed suicide. As a result of her earlier relationship with Julius Caesar, however, Egypt seems to have avoided the normal Roman despoliation of conquered lands. As Caesar had not let loose his troopers on Egypt, neither did Antony, nor even Octavion, who was constrained both by the popular memory of the honors that his stepfather, Julius Caesar, had heaped on his Egyptian lover and mother of his son and by the need to placate Egyptians who were fond of their queen. Had Cleopatra not taken a combative role, her country might have been spared the levies she and Antony made upon it. Furthermore, she herself might have survived, though a victorious Octavion would doubtless have slaughtered Caesarion lest he become a political threat.[24]

So the courtesies, the flattery, and the bribes had great utility, as well as limits. The Greeks were unable to oust the Romans with such measures or to prevent the Romans of the late republic from fighting destructive wars on Greek soil and at a terrible cost to the Greeks. These wars included that against Mithridates and the civil wars decided by the battles at Pharsalus, Philippi, and Actium.[25] Under certain circumstances, however, giving sexual pleasure was a more effective defense, as Cleopatra's Egypt learned to its great relief.

The experience of a century and a half as rulers of Greece did not lessen the attractions of foreign ways or ease Roman fears that their practical, blunt Roman culture was suffering corrosion from foreign, especially Greek, influences. Indeed, the Romans, especially after Julius Caesar's adventures in the arms of Cleopatra, shared Greek anxiety about alluring strangers and the pleasures of the flesh. They turned that fear back on the Greeks and other foreigners, not merely in the brutality of religious persecution but also in the literature dearest to their heart. The foremost literary expression of this unease was in the first book of the *Aeneid*, Vergil's epic celebration of the founding of Rome. Vergil's poem summoned up the mythical story of the Trojans, who suffered disaster by accepting a Greek gift. The few Trojans who survived set the stage for the founding of Rome, despite terrible opposition from brooding Juno, whose beauty Paris had slighted. Aeneas, whose stock would found Rome, reached Italy only after turning his back on that most beautiful of women, the widow Dido, founder of Carthage, and spurning her magnificent hospitality. To protect Aeneas, Venus had silently wounded Dido with a passionate love, a madness, for the young wandering Trojan. In the fourth book of the epic, Vergil had Aeneas turn aside momentarily from his duty to return Dido's love. Recalled to his duty and warned that he was in danger because women are always fickle and changeable, the grief-stricken Aeneas hastened his departure and left a shamed, distraught Dido to commit suicide.

By the Augustan age, when Vergil penned his epic to give the Romans a counterpart to Homer's work, to praise the new monarchy, and to lecture his countrymen on the evils of foreign ways, the upper classes of Rome were becoming thoroughly hellenized. Conservative Romans, filled with a sense of cultural inferiority, had good reason to be anxious about foreigners and their allure. The success of the Romans in expanding their empire into distant lands had proven expensive and corrosive. Not only had the republic and many Romans perished in civil wars between militarists who wanted to control the fruits of empire but as the poet Horace wrote in his *Epistles*, "captured Greece took her fierce victor captive and brought the arts into rustic Latium."[26]

As Rome expanded, Latin culture not only disintegrated along class lines, as noted above, but it also thinned out. There were simply too few Romans to teach by word or example the multitudes taken by Roman legions. Romans died in battle; Romans died in pestilences that racked Rome and other urban areas after the time of Christ; and Roman birthrates plummeted due to the reluctance of women to bear numerous children and perhaps also to environmental and sociological factors that especially affected the rich. To maintain distant frontiers or to extend the frontiers and capture more subjects, imperial Rome recruited more non-Romans as both ordinary soldiers and officers. They joined an imperial system that brutalized the subjects it already had, not least the crucial ones who lived in the border regions. The costs of imperial expansion fell especially heavily on them, for it was on the frontiers that most of Rome's soldiers and sailors were stationed. The more legions and fleets were present, the less people could afford to take on Roman ways, arguably the most important factor in the durability of the empire.[27]

It was the frontier region that posed the greatest threat to the Roman empire, not because one found threatening aliens there, but because one found there imperial Roman troops who, when deprived of their pay, fell rapaciously upon civilians and robbed them of the means to be Romans, or even drove them to revolt. It was there that one found would-be kingmakers. Indeed, throughout the empire the military became more and more rapacious, until one observer could write of "the peace-time war, one almost worse than the barbarian war and arising from the military's indiscipline and the officers' greed."[28] In sum, the bigger and more militarized the empire, the less Roman it was and the more alien and alienated its subjects, especially along the frontiers. Even had Roman militarists not thrown the empire into civil war on many occasions, the dynamics of the empire were such that militarism was killing the Roman empire. *Animus romanus* was killing and eventually killed *anima romana*.[29]

The Romans reached the apex of their empire around 70 A.D., just before the Jewish Rebellion. Up until that time, they had surrounded their empire with client states and kept them pliant with the flattery of honorific titles, bribes, and occasional armed support. Roman diplomats worked hard to make the network of client states work for the empire. When the Jewish zealots led their nation in a rebellion that threatened to inspire many other subject peoples, the Romans obsessively used their entire strategic reserve to crush the rebels. Whether the Romans intended to give the empire and its neighbors an object lesson in the gruesome fate of rebels or merely followed their normal operating procedure to its gruesome conclusion, the empire demonstrated the limits of its power. The clients soon thereafter became less pliant and more demanding. Disturbed by this turn of events, the Romans set out to absorb many of their restive clients, taking on the fatal responsibility of dealing directly with a host of new nations along the rim of the newly expanded empire.[30]

Expansion was greatest and most burdensome in the east. The foremost proponent of the doomed strategy was the bellicose emperor, Trajan. The overstretched empire now found that tribal chieftains who previously had gratefully accepted subsidies as rewards for good behavior now made good behavior dependent on subsidies. The Romans found themselves forced to pay more for good behavior.[31]

Abandonment of the buffer state system in favor of forward, fixed frontiers led to imperial overextension, loss of strategic flexibility, and a decline in fighting strength when the legions were moved from field camps into frontier cities. There the troops fell victim to the same civilized pleasures that had plagued Roman legionnaires in Spain and softened so many neighbors of the empire. Thereafter, the imperial forces and the empire itself fell victim to the Germans, Vandals, and other tribes from northern Europe. The Germans in particular had a superior agriculture and a less autocratic system. They were better organized and less savage than the Celts and tougher and less extended than the Romans. The Germans' base was solid, while the Romans, in some crucial respects like a Chinese dynasty, had hollowed out their empire by overextending it and making it dependent on a bloated, semi-foreign, and treacherous military establishment. Dependence on slavery weakened the Roman empire even more.

The northerners by no means succeeded all at once, just as the Romans did not swiftly fall. Faced with the threat from the northerners, the Romans set them against one another and tried to buy them off with land, titles, and material gifts. For centuries, the Roman strategy succeeded. They caught the leadership of tribe after tribe in a web of concessions and gift-giving, such as that marking the end of Caesar's Gallic war, as noted above. A century after Caesar, for example, the emperor Domitian used not only large sums of money but also technical aid in the form of artisans to placate the Dacians. The emperor Trajan grew apprehensive about payments to the Dacians, went to war against them in 102 A.D., and captured their king.[32]

In his *Agricola*, the great Roman historian, Tacitus, gives the best description of the Roman way of taking over a hostile nation by luring its leadership into a demoralizing Romanized urban life with retail stores, bathhouses, and wonderful banquets. Therein he describes the steps taken by his father-in-law, the Roman leader, Agricola, who pursued a course of action similar to that taken earlier by other Romans in Gaul. "The unsuspecting Britons spoke of such novelties as 'civilization', when in fact they were only a feature of their enslavement," wrote Tacitus.[33]

Tacitus was a moralist as well as an acute historian and observer. Just as nothing earned his scorn more easily than to fall victim to Roman entrapment, nothing seems to have stoked his admiration higher than the ability to repel Roman blandishments and aggression. In his *Germania*, he reflected on two centuries of Roman failure to conquer Germany and drew particular attention to German simplicity of life, lack of greed except for foreign loot, and refusal to accept any obligation to reciprocate when given a gift. Each of those characteristics, missing from Celtic society, was a formidable rampart against Rome's diplomatic snares. Along with a tradition exalting the brave, armed free man, and an ability on the part of some of their leaders to learn Roman weaknesses while studying Roman ways and to use that knowledge against the Romans, those ramparts withstood even terrible battlefield defeats by the forces of servile Rome.[34]

It is important to observe here that Roman payments to the Germans apparently did not result in a substantial loss of specie to the Germans. On the contrary, as in the case of Chinese payments to their neighbors, Roman silver fueled German purchases of the simpler goods offered in trade by the Romans. The plain-living Germans preferred silver to gold, because it was convenient for purchasing that quality of merchandise. Wartime disrupted this backflow of coinage into the empire and resulted in coin hoarding on the German side. This suggests that the Romans lost three ways from war: the cost of military operations against a plain living foe whose defeat offered little loot; some coinage given in tribute; and loss of the profits of trade.[35]

By the end of the third century A.D., traditional Roman diplomacy became less effective, not merely because it could not ensnare the Germans as effectively as it had the Celts but also because the empire was being steadily militarized in appearance and operation, with an attendant decline in resources. The militarists were steadily consuming one another and imperial resources as well in internal power struggles. Compounding that drain was the threat of Parthia in the east. Since the Roman strategy depended on a military core which grew less supple with time, every movement of troops to the eastern frontiers exposed the inherent weakness of the empire and attracted Germanic invasions. Imperial officers who were left behind had few resources with which to buy off the foreigners. Landed magnates and aristocrats contributed less and less to civic activities and imperial defense. The opulence of their lives was a great burden on the empire and ordinary individuals alike. By the fourth century A.D., the empire had taken on the additional burdens of building a magnificent second capital and an expensive Christian Church.

Against such a background of increasing demands on the wealth of society and the need to move resources from a wealthy East, where two-thirds of the taxes were raised to a beleaguered West, where two-thirds of the military operated, the decision to formally divide the empire in 395 A.D. proved fatal. Chester Starr notes of the fall of the empire in the west, that the western Romans no longer had the resources to follow "the old Roman custom of reenforcing diplomacy with bribes." Consequently, they were unable "to satisfy the Visigothic leader Alaric, who proceeded to take Rome in 410 A.D. and sack it for three days."[36] Subsequently, it fell to the clergy to treat with invaders and soften their blows. It was Pope Leo who secured from Gaiseric the agreement that in plundering Rome in 455 A.D. the Vandals would not rape or assault the Romans.[37]

The pressure on the population to support a half million soldiers and sailors was overwhelming. The expenditures on the military, coupled with the cost of supporting large numbers of magnates, never left much for buying peace or supporting the peasantry and educating it to Roman ways. Consequently, the shattering of the empire was all the more complete, splitting along the lines of unabsorbed and undigested tribal customs. The empire had proven to be an agglomeration of thousands of tribes, many of them as ready to pillage as the Roman empire had been to extort.[38]

NOTES

1. Robert B. Asprey, *War in the Shadows: The Guerrilla in History, Vol. 1* (Garden City, N.Y.: Doubleday & Co., 1975), pp. 16–30.

2. Stephen L. Dyson, *The Creation of the Roman Frontier* (Princeton, N.J.: Princeton University Press, 1985), pp. 13, 29. The susceptibility of Celtic leaders to bribery was known to and exploited by the Greek city of Massilia in Gaul as well. Ibid., p. 144.

3. Ibid., pp. 69–72.

4. Dyson, *The Creation of the Roman Frontier*, pp. 127–128; Chester G. Starr, *The Roman Empire 27 B.C.–A.D. 476: A Study in Survival* (New York: Oxford University Press, 1982), p. 80. Starr, ibid., pp. 21–22, 19, and 42, feels that Augustus Caesar made an unfortunate decision to stop expansion into Germany while, by contrast, Claudius was ill-advised to extend Roman rule over the rebellious Britons.

5. Ramsay MacMullen, *Enemies of the Roman Order: Treason, Unrest, and Alienation in the Empire* (Cambridge, Mass.: Harvard University Press, 1966), pp. 229–241, 53.

6. Alan Wardman, *Rome's Debt to Greece* (New York: St. Martin's Press, 1976), pp. xiv–xv.

7. J.V.D.P. Balsdon, *Romans and Aliens* (Chapel Hill: University of North Carolina Press, 1979), pp. 50, 38.

8. Athenaeus, *The Deipnosophists*, Vol. 5, trans. Charles Burton Gulick (Cambridge, Mass.: Harvard University Press; London: Heinemann, 1933), pp. 478–481.

9. Balsdon, *Romans and Aliens*, pp. 237–239, plays down the orgiastic aspects of Isis worship and notes that it set a high price on chastity.

10. MacMullen, *Enemies of the Roman Order*, pp. 219–221.

11. Wardman, *Rome's Debt to Greece*, pp. 1, 16. See also Balsdon, *Romans and Aliens*, pp. 38–50.

12. Wardman, *Rome's Debt to Greece*, pp. 8–9.

13. Ibid., pp. 16–17, 21.

14. Marcus Tullius Cicero, *De Senectute, De Amicitia, De Divinatione*, trans. William Armistead Falconer (Cambridge, Mass.: Harvard University Press; London: W. Heinemann, 1923), pp. 196–201; Wardman, *Rome's Debt to Greece*, pp. 36, 38.

15. Balsdon, *Romans and Aliens*, pp. 62–63.

16. John H. D'Arms, *Commerce and Social Standing in Ancient Rome* (Cambridge, Mass.: Harvard University Press, 1981), p. 21.

17. Balsdon, *Romans and Aliens*, p. 62.

18. Caius Julius Caesar, *The Gallic War*, trans. H.J. Edwards (Cambridge, Mass.: Harvard University Press; London: W. Heinemann, 1917), pp. 70–75.

19. D'Arms, *Commerce and Social Standing in Ancient Rome*, p. 33. Governmental support for commerce is surveyed in M. P. Charlesworth, *Trade-Routes and Commerce of the Roman Empire*, 2nd rev. ed. (Chicago: Ares, 1974), pp. 224–240.

20. Dyson, *The Creation of the Roman Frontier*, pp. 54, 132.

21. Caius Julius Caesar, *The Gallic War*, pp. 2–3, 182–183, 348–351.

22. Ibid., pp. 470–471.

23. Ibid., pp. 582–583.

24. T. Rice Holmes, *The Architect of the Roman Empire* (Oxford: Clarendon Press, 1928; reprint, New York: AMS Press, 1977), pp. 137, 142–171.

25. Wardman, *Rome's Debt to Greece*, pp. 26–30.

26. Ibid., p. ix.

27. On the "really predatory nature of the military," which Ramsay MacMullen found to be obvious in all regions and centuries of the Principate, see his *Corruption and the Decline of Rome* (New Haven, Conn. and London: Yale University Press, 1988), pp. 129–132. On a common culture as the necessary foundation of the empire, see Dyson, *The Creation of the Roman Frontier*, p. 262, wherein Dyson makes the same point somewhat more broadly: "In Sardinia, as elsewhere, the

creation of a frontier during the Republic was not just a matter of military pacification and tribal decimation. It involved building roads, establishing settlements, and most important, cultivating a Mediterranean high-culture life that would provide the basic support for Roman rule."

28. MacMullen, *Corruption and the Decline of Rome*, pp. 131–132, 191–194.

29. Peter Garnsey and Richard Saller, *The Roman Empire: Economy, Society, and Culture* (Berkeley: University of California Press, 1987), pp. 83–103, argue that the size of the empire gave a large enough tax base to keep tax rates relatively low, except in Egypt. Still, by their own account, non-Roman cultural luminaries in the empire came primarily from areas such as Gaul and Spain, which by then had no legions present, or from Africa, which was not heavily defended. Ibid., pp. 186–189.

30. Edward N. Luttwak, *The Grand Strategy of the Roman Empire from the First Century A.D. to the Third* (Baltimore: Johns Hopkins University Press, 1976), pp. 32–37, 108–117. Starr, *The Roman Empire 27 B.C.–A.D. 476*, p. 121, feels, contrary to Luttwak, that the obliteration of the Jews at Massada was merely the consequence of Roman generals following standard operating procedure. In light of Dio's analysis in his *History of Rome*, that the Jewish rebels were inspiring restlessness throughout the empire, I believe that Luttwak is on stronger ground. See Casseius Dio Cocceianus, *Dio's Roman History, Vol. 8*, with an English translation by Earnest Cary, Ph.D., on the basis of the version of Herbert Baldwin Foster (Cambridge, Mass.: Harvard University Press; London: W. Heinemann, 1925), pp. 446–453.

31. Luttwak, *The Grand Strategy of the Roman Empire from the First Century A. D. to the Third*, pp. 115–116.

32. Mortimer Wheeler, *Rome beyond the Imperial Frontiers* (Westport, Conn.: Greenwood Press, 1971, orig. pub. 1954), p. 10.

33. Ibid., pp. 19–21. See also Garnsey and Saller, *The Roman Empire*, pp. 17–19.

34. Dyson, *The Creation of the Roman Frontier*, p. 68.

35. Wheeler, *Rome beyond the Imperial Frontiers*, pp. 63–68.

36. Starr, *The Roman Empire 27 B.C.–A.D. 476*, pp. 167–168.

37. Ibid., p. 173.

38. MacMullen, *Enemies of the Roman Order*, p. 215.

4

The Glittering Diplomacy
of Byzantium

When debilitated Rome fell to the Vandals in 455 A.D., the end of the Roman empire in the West was little more than two decades in the future. But Constantinople, founded in 330 A.D. by Constantine, lived on for nearly a thousand more years as the capital of a Roman East known as Byzantium. Its subjects, though Greek in culture, called themselves "Romans" and referred to their capital simply as "The City." Constantinople was the beacon of a Christianized Graeco-Roman civilization. Until it too fell to invaders, the great city by the Straits of the Bosporus survived wave after wave of crisis, many caused or exacerbated by dictatorship, irredentism, military insubordination, religious zealotry, and the oppressive behavior of both bureaucrats and, especially, of landed magnates. The key means of survival was diplomacy, and Byzantine diplomats depended on the pleasure given by the high culture of their great city as one of their most powerful tools.

Had Byzantium been more faithful to the art of diplomacy and still less inclined than it was to the art of war, it might still exist. But it periodically embarked on military crusades that greatly weakened it and on two occasions threatened its own survival. As Owen Lattimore noted of the Chinese, so in the case of the Byzantines, imperial expansion was illusory and carried with it the seeds of its own undoing. Like Southern Song trying to regain north China, Byzantium crippled itself through irredentist attempts to regain the lost western portions of the old Roman empire. The cost of Emperor Leo's unsuccessful attempts in 468 and 470 A.D. to retake northern Africa from the Vandals staggered the government and made it difficult to pay the army. Disgruntled generals struggled for power, threatening Emperor Leo. The year 471 A.D. was a watershed year and for nearly a half century, until 520 A.D., "the empire experienced one of the most active periods of abortive military unrest in its history. Leo, in fact, had to buy an expensive peace in 473 A.D. from the Ostrogothic King Theodoric Strabo, who had allied with some of Leo's rebellious Gothic soldiers."[1]

Straining under the cost of maintaining so many soldiers, the empire had barely escaped the worst of the internal military unrest when it suffered the Emperor Justinian's (527–565 A.D.) irredentist attempts to recapture the lost western portions of the old Roman empire. To take but one example, Justinian's war against the Ostrogoths in Italy lasted twenty years. His militaristic dream of grandeur was a heavy burden for the Byzantines but a deadly nightmare for the Italians. In words that might have been written by Tacitus, Louis Brehier, the great historian of Byzantium, wrote, "Italy had been recovered, and Justinian prided himself on having saved it from tyranny and established stable peace there in the Pragmatic Sanction by which he reorganized its administration. But the picture of Italy painted by contemporaries shows it emerging from this war devastated, depopulated, and lastingly impoverished. The countryside was deserted, works of art, roads, aqueducts and dykes were in ruins, and the towns had been decimated by plague."[2]

Having committed his armies elsewhere, Justinian hoped to defend the Danube frontier by a combination of static defense and clever intrigue, so he built fortresses, lines of fortification, and towns and castles from the Danube through Thrace and into Greece. He also provoked "the peoples settled north of the River Danube or in Noricum into conflict among themselves: the Lombards against the Gepids of the Hungarian Plain; the Utigur Huns east of the Sea of Azov against the Kutrigur Huns between the Don and the Dniester, who were allies of the Gepids; and lastly a newly-arrived people, the Avars, who were really Uighur Turks, . . . against all the other Danube peoples."[3]

The imperial heartland soon paid heavily in blood for this bellicosity and mischievous intrigue. By dispersing his country's forces, defeating states that might otherwise have been buffers, provoking its neighbors to fight among themselves, and draining its treasury, Justinian opened Byzantium to attack by the Bulgars, Slavs, Huns, and Persians. Before they were defeated, war bands of the first three peoples had devastated Greece and the Balkans and reached the gates of Constantinople. When the Persians were beaten by an expensive counteroffensive led by Heraclius early in the next century, Byzantium had few resources to use against the Arabs, who were emerging as the empire's most formidable foe.

Byzantium's strain of militarism was nothing new. It had inherited from Rome this crucial internal political problem: how to maintain a military establishment large enough to protect the interests of the empire, but not large enough to threaten the state. As Walter E. Kaegi, Jr., observed in his study of Byzantine military unrest from 471 to 843 A.D., "According to tradition, ever since the early Republic Rome had experienced difficulties arising from the ability of soldiers to exert pressure on the government, which needed military manpower. Byzantium inherited from Rome this tradition and historical record of seditions, civil wars, ambitious and rebellious generals, and violent usurpations of the imperial throne."[4]

Compounding irredentism and militarism was religious fanaticism. Terrible divisions over theological issues split Christianity in the East. One of the dividing issues was the role of icons and other representations of religious significance. Those against representation of religious figures, the iconoclasts or image breakers, made up a large part of the Christian communities of North Africa, Egypt, and Syria and felt little loyalty to the iconophiles who clustered around Constantinople's ruling group. Byzantium needed wholehearted support from its iconoclastic subjects on the fringe of the empire to fend off the Arabs who were filled with iconoclastic Islamic zeal. Christian iconoclasts were more willing, if not eager, to be subjects of the Arabs than of the hated iconophiles.

Thus weakened by fanatical irredentism, always expensive militarism, and religious fanaticism, Byzantium lost North Africa, Egypt, Syria, and Armenia to the Arabs and most of Italy to the Lombards. Consequently, the character of the empire became more Greek, still more militarized, and more superstitious.[5] Relations with the neighboring Bulgars deteriorated into fruitless warfare that ended temporarily only with the death of the Bulgar khan Krum in 814 A.D. as he prepared a second attack on Constantinople. Rather than seeking a wider peace, however, Byzantium, under Basil I (d. 867 A.D.), an arriviste Macedonian stable boy, went to war against the Arabs and expanded almost to Jerusalem. It also reasserted itself in Italy.

The subsequent conversion of the Bulgars to Christianity later in the ninth century A.D. and the education of the young Bulgarian royal prince, Symeon, in the City might have been lasting grounds for peace on the Balkan frontier. But rather than enjoy the benefits from an expansion of their culture and trade, the Byzantines decided to make the highly successful

Bulgarian commercial operations in the empire difficult and dangerous. Symeon, who had been so dazzled by the splendors of the Sacred Palace that even after his ascent of the Bulgar throne "he dreamed of nothing less than his own coronation as basileus" (emperor), seized on the threat to Bulgarian trade as a reason for war. To deter him, the Byzantines engaged the Hungarians to fall upon and devastate Bulgaria. Symeon beat them off only with great difficulty. Then he turned on the Byzantines and threw them back behind the walls of the City itself. At that point, the Byzantines sued for peace and reached a reasonable agreement with him in 896 A.D. The difficulty of breaching the City's massive fortifications and the threat from the Hungarians tempered but did not eradicate Symeon's desire for revenge.[6]

The Byzantines soon became caught up in another of their internal power struggles and reneged on their promises of a modest tribute to Symeon. Empress Zoe compounded this stinginess by canceling the treaty with Bulgaria. This provoked a brutal three-year war (914–917 A.D.) in which Symeon crushed both the Byzantines and the Pechenegs, a nomadic people engaged to war upon the Bulgarians. Symeon fought his way to the City but turned away at the sight of the ramparts and marched off to devastate Greece. More Byzantine power struggles encouraged the ambitious Symeon to hope that he might ascend to the Byzantine throne or have his daughter marry the royal prince. Frustrated, Symeon launched another devastating war against Byzantium. The Byzantines countered by bribing Prince Paul of Serbia to revolt against his Bulgar overlord. Symeon crushed Paul and his troops. Symeon needed a fleet to take the City, so he allied with the Fatimids of Africa, but the Byzantines captured the Arab ambassadors and won them over to their side. Then in 924 A.D., the fifth year of the war, Symeon appeared with his army in the shadow of the City that so dazzled him and inexplicably demanded and got a truce, agreeing to turn over some places on the Black Sea in exchange for a small tribute and a few presents. Symeon never turned back those places. To the dismay of the Greeks, he went home and styled himself "basileus and autocrator of the Bulgarians and the Greeks." The Byzantines protested. The pope, however, confirmed Symeon's title and, in addition, conferred the title of patriarch on the archbishop of Bulgaria.[7]

After Symeon's death in 927 A.D., the Byzantines went back to their standard diplomatic practice and successfully bought peace from the Bulgars by marrying a princess royal to his son Peter. She changed her name to Eirene (Peace) as a symbol of a new era in Bulgarian-Byzantine relations. As part of the peace agreement, there was a border adjustment near Thessalonica in exchange for the return of some Byzantine cities on the Gulf of Burgas, the conferral of the title *basileus* on the Bulgarian king, and an agreement to give Bulgarian ambassadors precedence over all other ambassadors. The treaty left the Byzantines free to deal with their archenemy, the Arabs, and the Bulgars free to contend with theirs, the Hungarians.[8]

Rather than enjoying the fruits of peace, the Byzantines now turned to a relentless war to reconquer all of the area that had been lost to the empire over the previous three centuries. It abandoned its relatively inexpensive regional army organization, known as the thematic army, and turned to a professional army structure. Soon it was the dominant military power in Christian Europe and the Middle East. Its success at manufacturing and selling luxury goods and extracting even more taxes from an already overtaxed peasantry gave it, temporarily, the means to be so aggressive.[9] Not only did the empire push into Arab-dominated lands, but fifty years of peace with the Bulgarians went by the boards as the Byzantines struggled with them and the Russians for the Danube. It is instructive that the Byzantines initially paid the Russians to attack the Bulgarians. Only with great difficulty were the Byzantines able to defeat the Russians and annex part of Bulgaria. Peace with the Russians came about in a typical Byzantine fashion. In 988 A.D., Emperor Basil II had secured his own position on the throne with the aid of 6,000 Russian warriors dispatched by Russian Prince Vladimir in exchange for the promise of the hand of his sister, Anna Porphyrogenita, and assistance in converting his people to Orthodox Christianity. When Basil II delayed in dispatching Anna, Vladimir took the city of Cherson on the Black Sea and returned it only upon Anna's arrival. Further Byzantine expansion into Bulgaria took place during the nearly half-century reign of Basil II (d. 1025 A.D.), who warred against the Bulgarians for nearly twenty years, savagely crushed them, and incorporated them into the Byzantine empire.

Although Basil II's reign was one of the peaks of Byzantine imperialism, the ascent to that peak entailed gruesome domestic and international measures that would weaken Byzantium enough to send it into a decline from which it never recovered. To amass the wealth necessary to expand the borders of the empire and beautify the capital city, Basil II nipped the growing provincial market economies and ground down the free peasantry as well as the magnates until forced during the last two years of his reign to let the taxes on the pitiful peasantry go uncollected. But the conquest of the Bulgarians did not bring much wealth into the empire. Indeed, the Bulgars initially paid taxes in kind because their country was so poor. Furthermore, having lost Bulgaria as a buffer state, the Byzantines now had to defend the Balkans against invaders from the steppes. The cost of imperial defense would rise still further because Basil II, through force and diplomacy, also annexed the Armenian principalities and lost those crucial buffers against the Turks. And by taking in the Armenian homeland of the heretical Monophysite Christians, Basil II also introduced a highly divisive religious aspect into his Orthodox Christian empire, an empire whose leadership was morbidly threatened by people and things non-Greek.[10]

As Michael Angold observed of this period of expansion, "Byzantium, like so many other imperial powers, was always at its most vulnerable when a period of conquest and expansion was coming to an end. It took time to realize that the aggressive foreign policy inherited from Basil II had little to recommend it. The cost of maintaining the Empire on a permanent war footing was becoming exorbitant and the gains were negligible." Arnold Toynbee noted of Basil II's war of annihilation against the Bulgarian resistance movement that it was a replay of Justinian's war to the death with the Ostrogoths in Italy. "Once again, the Empire's already heavily taxed resources were being overstrained for the sake of achieving a conquest that was both unnecessary and eventually untenable. Basil II's war with Tsar Samuel left Basil with no margin to spare for any other purpose. He let the East Roman Navy decay. Venice was the beneficiary."[11]

Basil II's immediate successor, Constantine VIII, sparked a peasant rebellion in mainland Greece and drove the Anatolian peasantry off their farms by trying to squeeze five years of taxes out of them in three years. His successor, Romanus III Argyros, aided the poor but abandoned diplomacy and squandered Byzantine wealth in conquests beyond the Euphrates and in vain attempts to conquer Aleppo in Syria, Egypt, and Sicily. His successor, Michael IV the Paphlagonian (1034–1041 A.D.), tried to repair the damage to the state treasury by exacting money taxes from the Bulgarians and merely sparked a rebellion there in 1040 A.D. Constantine IX Monomachos (1042–1055 A.D.) adopted a defensive posture at the frontiers, emphasized diplomacy, and in the case of mass starvation in Egypt, sent relief supplies of corn. But Constantine bungled the disbandment of some Byzantine troops and set off a military revolt. The frequent shifts back and forth between military and diplomatic approaches to foreign affairs undermined the effectiveness of Byzantine diplomacy. The requisite steadiness was quite lacking.[12]

The military victories of Basil II and his successors, though assisted by a superior military organization and technology, including the dreaded Greek fire, proved to be short-lived. In its struggle with the lay and ecclesiastical magnates over the wealth of the countryside, the state lost the free peasantry as a source of the revenues and soldiers needed for diplomacy and defense. Byzantium was falling into feudalism just when the Normans appeared to strip away the empire's southern Italian provinces and two groups of Turks, including the Seljuks, appeared in 1081 A.D. at the gates of Constantinople ready to crush the rest of the failing empire. Nonetheless, the empire survived because the newly crowned emperor, Alexius Comnenus, seized and melted down or sold many church treasures to buy the military services of a third Turkish people who helped drive off the other Turks.[13] There is no more dramatic example in the history of diplomacy of the power of money. Money, bribes if you will, had saved Byzantium. There is no other explanation for its survival at that juncture. The empire would continue on for more than three and a half centuries, longer than a typical Chinese dynasty.

A decade later, Emperor Alexius I Comnenus used pleasure to recruit allies in an attempt to regain Byzantium's frontier on the Danube River from an erstwhile ally, a Turkish people known as the Pechenegs. He wooed the leaders of another Turkish group, the Cumans. A splendid banquet for them was apparently the deciding factor, and the Cumans turned on the Pechenegs and smashed them in battle. Within a few years, however, the Cumans turned on the Byzantines, who finally overcame them piecemeal when they broke into raiding parties.[14]

Byzantium flourished until the late twelfth century, when Manuel I Comnenus weakened it by alienating Western Christendom and alarming its neighbors with an aggressive revanchism, the Song dynasty disease of trying to restore old imperial boundaries. By permitting the exploitation of the participants in the second crusade (1146–1148 A.D.) through the sale of adulterated provisions and the issue of debased coinage, he squandered most of the little sympathy Byzantium had in the West. Western Christians changed their opinion of the Byzantine empire. Before the crusade, Peter the Venerable, abbot of Cluny, the great western monastery, wrote of the Byzantine empire, "Standing at the mid-point of east, west, and north, it overawed the east, subdued the north, and defended the west." After the failure of the crusade, Peter and others in the West wanted to take revenge on Byzantium for the failure of the crusade.[15] Venice, which long had had a near monopoly of trade between Constantinople and the West and had supplied the Byzantine empire with the bulk of its naval forces, might yet have stood with the Byzantines had not Manuel decided to offset Venice's role by extending similar trading privileges to Pisa and Genoa. As Veneto-Byzantine relations deteriorated, Manuel took the fateful step in March 1171 A.D. of expelling all Venetians from the empire and confiscating their goods. Venice would later have its revenge by steering the Fourth Crusade against Byzantium. By his attacks on Egypt (1169 A.D.) and Turkish Anatolia (1176 A.D.), Manuel I Comnenus wasted the empire's internal resources. Had he not so squandered the City's political and financial resources, it might not have fallen victim to the soldiery of the Fourth Crusade in 1204 A.D., a blow from which Byzantium never fully recovered.

After the fall of Constantinople to the crusaders, many decades passed before the Greeks regained control of the City in 1261 A.D. Venice took over the riches of Crete, and Genoa those of Chios. Under the circumstances, Byzantine diplomats suffered terrible handicaps. The leaders of the various fragments of the empire fought among themselves. Their struggles were so bitter that they sparked a democratic rebellion among the long-suffering imperial subjects in Thessalonike. Most of the empire's resources were lost to other states, wasted in internal power struggles, or hoarded by the church and thus unavailable to diplomats. There was no Alexius Comnenus to seize the church's gold and save the City. The Orthodox Church's doctrinal inflexibility also greatly hampered the emperors and their diplomatic corps.

Byzantine diplomats did score one major coup during these years of decline, the Sicilian Vespers of 1282 A.D., a revolt of the people of Sicily against French rule. Byzantium had been fighting to regain southern Greece from the French. The French in turn began planning a crusade to be launched against Byzantium in 1283 A.D. They started to amass a fleet in Sicily, where they ruled in a brutal fashion; they also called on the Venetians for ships. Byzantine Emperor Michael VIII secured help from his son-in-law, the King of Hungary, from the Mamluk Sultan of Egypt, from the Khan of the Golden Horde, as well as from an old enemy of the French, Peter III of Aragon. Most importantly, Byzantine spies spread gold among the discontented Sicilians, who rose up in March 1282 A.D. and destroyed the French fleet. In August, assisted with more Byzantine gold, Peter III of Aragon arrived with a military force and expelled the French.

Michael VIII did not live long to savor the triumph. In December 1282 A.D. he died, having failed to unify Byzantium politically or religiously. Some of his attempts to unify Greek and Latin Christianity and deflect Latin political pressure had alienated his Greek subjects. Torn from within and beset by strong enemies, the empire staggered along, watching more and more of its subjects willingly become Turkish subjects and Muslims rather than suffer longer the oppression of the Byzantine state and church. Byzantine diplomacy relied more and more on marital alliances. To buy off the leader of the Serbs, an increasingly dangerous neighbor, Emperor

Andronicus II Paleologus, offered the hand of an imperial princess, his niece, the widow of the king of Trebizond. But she refused to leave the luxury of the City. So Andronicus gave his five-year-old daughter, Simonis, instead, along with title to Byzantine land that the Serbian had captured. The Serbian, Uros II Milutin, fell under the influence of his new mother-in-law, Eirene. In that same period, he tried to draw in the King of Lesser Armenia by having his son and heir marry the king's sister in 1296 A.D. Diplomacy, however, was unable to overcome all of the failings of the empire, even when the Mongols overran the Ottoman Turks in 1402 A.D. Indeed, by this time, Greek diplomats seemed to have lost their touch and unwittingly assisted in the rebirth of the Ottoman empire. It is not clear whether the Emperor Manuel II's warm friendship with the Turkish Sultan Muhammad contributed to the blunders, but it did shield Manuel from Turkish retribution for his actions against the Turks. Upon the accession of a new Sultan, Murad II, the pleasant shield of friendship was finally lost, and what was left of the empire became a Turkish vassal and withered until the Turks captured the City in 1453 A.D.

The fall to the Turks of a diminished and weakened Constantinople set off a wave of consternation in the Christian West. The reasons for the fall of Byzantium amount to the familiar pattern of an adventurous and a wasteful dictatorship, a rebellious military composed in large part of foreigners, an oppressed and a disaffected peasantry, and an expensive church which drained away men and money from the government and civil society. If we look to the twin Greek and Roman cultural roots of the empire, it is possible to see Greek divisiveness and superstition combining with Roman love of glory and military parasitism. Still, the empire lasted a millennium, because it had a much more wealthy base than did the Roman West. On this base it could build a strong military and, more importantly, a clever and an effective diplomatic corps which made resort to military action generally unnecessary.

Byzantine diplomacy was a marvel built upon centuries of Greek and Roman experiences in dealing with outsiders. It also combined powerful Greek and Roman cultural traits. When not weakened by military adventurers, like Justinian or, centuries later, Manuel Comnenus, who were eager to recapture the gory glory of Rome, or by religious zealots, Byzantine foreign policy was truly the shield of the state.

Like the Romans, the Byzantines normally preferred clever diplomacy to military action. They studied their neighbors closely, keeping notes on the most influential families, on "what presents pleased them best, which of their sentiments or interests might be most usefully cultivated, and what political or economic relations might be established with them." Thus evolved a real "science of governing barbarians."[16]

At the heart of Byzantine diplomacy was the belief that every person could be won over by money. The Byzantine rulers' "crudest, simplest, and most direct way of influencing foreign nations was by means of money," a way that Diehl tells us "they used indiscriminately and sometimes unwisely, in and out of season."[17] It ought to be no surprise that the Byzantine Greeks believed in the efficacy of gifts and bribes. As we have seen, their Greek history told them that gifts and bribes worked well; Roman history reinforced the lesson; success proved it time and again. Gifts and bribes were as useful to Justinian, who kept all of his barbarian king neighbors in his pay, as they were to Alexius Comnenus six centuries later in buying off Latin crusaders. They took varying forms, including the terribly expensive and ultimately crippling self-exemption from taxes that was granted to Venetian and later Pisan and Genoan traders within the Byzantine empire.

Like the Chinese and the Romans, the Byzantines also sought the goodwill of foreign princes in other, less expensive ways, such as the conferral of honorific titles. Like the Chinese, they also bestowed wives and ceremonial robes on neighbors whose support they desired. Marriage alliances were an important element of Byzantine diplomacy. For political, economic, and aesthetic reasons, foreign leaders often sought the hand of noble Byzantine women in marriage. So Charlemagne, newly crowned king of the Romans in 800 A.D. by a grateful Pope Leo, whom he had restored to the papal throne, sought to legitimate his new title in the East by marrying Eirene, the dowager Byzantine empress. Eirene inclined to the marriage. European history might have been quite different had it not been for the strenuous objections of Aetius, one of her eunuch advisers. While he waited on word of his long-distance courtship, Charlemagne put off preparing an attack on Sicily, a Byzantine possession.[18]

Noble Byzantine women also brought rich dowries to their new homes and, typically, the resplendence of a very beautiful woman, for the Byzantines deliberately chose beautiful women as royal wives. Beauty was indeed the only requisite for a Byzantine queen. Whatever their origins (Khazars, singers, cooks, prostitutes, and other entertainers all assumed the purple), empresses were expected to be beautiful and to have very attractive daughters who would make good marriage alliances. Thus when the first Comnenian empress, the very beautiful Eirene Doukaina, sent out for a young woman for her son to marry, she gave orders that the candidates would have to be virgins of a certain height, figure, age, and standard of beauty.[19]

In whatever form, the gifts were cunningly calculated to win favor from chosen neighbors while setting their neighbors against them. "Divide and conquer" was always a maxim influencing Byzantine generosity and all other aspects of its foreign policy. Looking at the grand sweep of Byzantium's millennium, Guerdan observes that, "The aim was not to beat one's enemies but to divide them; at various times she [Byzantium] set Venice against the Normans, the Italian cities against Frederick Barbarossa, Germany against France and the Kingdom of Sicily, Armenians against Arabs, and Russians against Bulgarians."[20]

Where such manipulation led to bloodshed among outsiders, the survivors might, as they did in Justinian's time, cross over the border battled hardened and eager to recoup their fortunes by looting and pillaging the empire. Then bands of Slavs, Bulgars, and Huns devastated the empire from the Adriatic to the walls of Constantinople, putting Greece to fire and sword. The Byzantines sorrowfully reaped what their too-clever, violence-prone leader had sown.

The Byzantines carefully managed all visits by foreign ambassadors to reinforce in their guests the sense of wealth, cultural attainment, and unity of the empire. From the moment ambassadors arrived at the imperial frontier and were officially received by high civilian and military officials, they were engaged in a carefully calibrated welcome and exchange of gifts. Similar well-planned ceremonies took place in major cities all along the way to the capital. Once in the capital, the Byzantines enveloped the official visitors in court rituals and banquet ceremonies and in tours of the most impressive parts of the city and its fortifications, all designed to impress them.[21]

To the unsophisticated, Byzantine court ceremony was indeed awe inspiring. The richly dressed emperor presented himself as a god, as Jesus Christ triumphant. As Rene Guerdan remarked, "His receptions were not audiences, but revelations. He did not merely make an appearance, he manifested himself."[22] Gilded automata in the shape of birds and lions making appropriate songs and roars greeted visitors who looked up from multiple prostrations to see the emperor raised high above them on a mechanically elevated throne. The theatrics, which included prostrations before the curtained throne and the raising of the throne with a baldachino over it, trace back to the court ceremonies of the Persian King Darius, as we know from the great relief of the treasury of Xerxes in Persepolis.[23] But they did not always produce the desired effect. More sophisticated envoys might remain detached from the spectacle. The tenth-century Italian bishop and envoy, Liudprand, for example, wrote that he was "moved neither by terror nor admiration, since I had learned much about all these things from men who knew them well."[24]

Official guests at Byzantine state banquets held in their honor found that the protocol was rigidly defined. Most of the other foreign ambassadors in Constantinople and most of the high officials attended the state banquets. Ambassadors took seats that reflected the current importance of their country to Constantinople, rather than, as in China, the history of relationships between their country and China. And unlike his Chinese counterpart, the Byzantine emperor ate with his guests. That made the occasion a religious one, so there were also specifically religious readings. To underscore the seriousness of such quasi-religious occasions, there were severe penalties for violation of the ritual, including decapitation for dropping a plate or blinding for seeing one dropped. There is no record of a noble or a foreign ambassador, however, suffering such penalties. The food and wine were plentiful, though not as numerous in kind as the Chinese court laid out. The final course was fruit, served in three baskets mechanically lowered from the ceiling and moved along past the guests. Musicians, mimes, dancers, Hindu jugglers, and Chinese acrobats entertained. And so that important guests would have something to take away from the table, the hosts passed out to them and their retainers handsome tips, gifts of money.[25]

The effect of a Byzantine state banquet could be overpowering, even on a hostile person such as Odo of Deuil, the French chronicler of the Second Crusade, who accompanied King Louis to a lavish banquet thrown by Manuel I Comnenus in Louis' honor on the feast day of St. Denis, patron saint of the French in the year 1147–1148 A.D. Odo concluded that, "No one could understand the Greeks without having had experience of them or without being endowed with prophetic inspiration."[26]

Formal religious ceremony in a church setting might supplement court ceremony. What some consider the most decisive event in early Russian history, the conversion of Prince Vladimir to Christianity in 988–989 A.D., which was followed by the baptism of his Kievan people in the Dnieper River, stemmed from a visit by Greek clergy to Kiev and a debate over the selection of a religion by Vladimir. The debate spawned official fact-finding tours, including a visit to Constantinople by an official Russian group seeking to compare Greek religion to what they had seen of Islam and of Western Christianity. They reported back to their prince that the beauty and splendor of the Greek churches and religious ceremonies were indescribably beautiful. They told their Prince, "[W]e knew not whether we were in heaven or on earth. . . . We know only that God dwells there among men, and their service is fairer than the ceremonies of other nations. For we cannot forget that beauty. Every man, after tasting something sweet, is afterward unwilling to accept that which is bitter, and therefore we cannot dwell longer here."[27]

The Byzantines included in their official hospitality tours of beautiful churches, luxurious palaces, opulent bazaars, and strong ramparts to reinforce that awe in the visitors. The official courtesies were carefully matched to the importance of the visitors, who were closely hedged about and their movements very restricted. Nonetheless, the squalid aspects of Constantinople did not escape the eyes of the sharp-eyed official visitor, such as Odo of Deuil in the reign of Manuel I Comnenus (1143–1180 A.D.), who observed how "the wealthy overshadow the streets with buildings and leave these dirty, dark places to the poor and travellers."[28]

The aim of the official hospitality was to have the visitors leave Byzantium well rewarded, properly dazzled, carrying a treaty favorable to Byzantine interests, and, if possible, accompanied by some Orthodox monks. These last would spread the influence of Byzantium in another way.

As for diplomatic negotiations themselves, they generally concerned economic issues arising from Constantinople's control of two sea straits. The negotiations took place in the imperial palace and followed a protocol that dated back to the late antique period. Having presented valid ambassadorial credentials, later deposited with any written agreement concluded, and distributed letters of introduction from their sovereign to almost all influential Byzantine government officials, foreign ambassadors would attempt in discussions with a high Byzantine official to reach a preliminary agreement in accordance with their written instructions. Having done that and sworn to it in the presence of the emperor, they would then sign and seal a draft of the agreement including their oath; thereupon the emperor would order the treaty to be prepared in both languages. At a subsequent ceremony, he would sign the two copies and give one to the ambassadors to take home in the company of a Byzantine legation. Upon their arrival home, the foreign heads of state had to swear to the treaty in the presence of the Byzantine envoys for the treaty to be binding on both sides. Much of this diplomatic protocol was adopted by Venice and then by the great western states, and it has survived to this day.[29]

There was another set of official visitors whom the Byzantines sought to impress with an eye to winning their allegiance—foreign prisoners of war. In greeting a triumphal army and its general, the Byzantines decorated their entire city with bunting, mobilized all of the city people to show off their silver and gold wares and paintings from their balconies, and filled the air with incense to mark the special nature of the occasion and also to demonstrate the wealth of the city and its people to the vanquished. After greeting the victorious general in his hour of triumph, the emperor would ritually put his foot on the head and his lance on the throat of the leader of the vanquished, while the other prisoners were thrown face down in the dirt of the Circus. Then the Byzantine policy of generosity took effect, and the emperor offered the wealth of the empire to the defeated leader and his officers. He gave them estates, a place at court, and the freedom of the city. If Muslim, they could attend a mosque; if they converted to Christianity, there was no limit on their social, and hence political, mobility. It was a clever policy and generally highly effective.[30]

There were dangerous aspects to Byzantine diplomacy. Proverbially beautiful Byzantine princesses were much sought after as wives by foreign rulers. But once given in marriage, the princesses provided those same foreign rulers with an excuse to meddle in Byzantine politics. Tax exemptions given to foreign merchants brought Constantinople some immediate advantage but eventually put Byzantine traders at such a disadvantage that Byzantium lost much of its merchant marine and was destabilized by anti-foreign sentiments that from time to time flared into deadly riots. These tax exemptions cost the state a great deal of money, while they opened up economic opportunities for landed magnates who exported foodstuffs to Italy and spent the wealth thus gained in struggles with the central government. If too rich, gifts could enrich an enemy enough to make it a stronger foe. And, as in the cases of China and Rome, bribes and favors could stir up voracious greed on the part of neighbors.

The very fineness of Byzantine foreign policy sometimes worked against it, perhaps even combining with some other Byzantine trait to further endanger a policy. The case of the marriage alliance between Byzantium and Germany at the outset of Manuel I Comnenus's reign is an example of how incessant political recalculation and a practical love of beauty nearly made an enemy of Germany at a critical time. Constantinople was losing Sicily and its Italian possessions to the Normans of Sicily and seemed to need German help against the Normans. In 1140 A.D., the Byzantines sent off a delegation to Germany with the proposal of a marriage alliance, but by the summer of 1142 A.D., when the rather plain Bertha of Sulzbach, sister-in-law of German Emperor Conrad III, arrived to marry Manuel, the Byzantines were having second thoughts and wanted to explore a rapprochement with the Normans. Moreover, Manuel now found aesthetic and social reasons for postponing or canceling the marriage. Bertha, who refused to slather herself in the Byzantine style with cosmetics, certainly did not meet the minimum standard for a Byzantine queen, that of personal beauty. So Manuel delayed marrying Bertha and at the end of 1144 A.D. sent off another diplomatic mission to Germany to improve the terms of the alliance. This delay only enraged the German emperor. Finally, the marriage was consummated, on slightly better terms, and the threat from the Normans was neutralized.[31]

The calculating, often indirect, nature of Byzantine foreign policy not only led to delays that exasperated allies but also eroded the sense of trust that could have led to smoother relations between Byzantium and the West, or for that matter, other neighbors. Contemporaries saw Byzantine foreign policy as all too crafty and guided only by reason of state. Odo of Deuil observed correctly that the Byzantines "are of the opinion that anything which is done for the Sacred Empire cannot be judged treachery."[32]

The Byzantines were aware that there were dangerous elements in their diplomatic style, but whether at home or abroad, the principles of pomp and generosity, designed to demonstrate that overwhelming resources were available to the nation, guided diplomatic thinking. As an illustration of this, we turn to a sixth-century author of a Byzantine treatise on strategy who called for generosity in receiving envoys. He went on to caution his compatriots against drawing the attention of envoys of nations superior in size or courage to Byzantium's wealth or the beauty of its women. Instead, he would point out to them the "number of our men, the polish of our weapons, and the height of our walls." The strategist expected that Byzantine envoys would be religious, free of a criminal past, intelligent, courageous and eager to serve. Furthermore, in the presence of those to whom they have been sent, "the envoys would appear gracious, truly noble, and generous to the extent of their powers." Indeed, the strategist singled out for criticism an anonymous envoy who had held back official gifts when he discovered that a neighboring state thought to be friendly was not. The strategist was of the opinion that the tight-fisted envoy would have done better to present at least some of the gifts to mollify the enemy. In that way, "[w]ithout seeming to enrich the enemy, he could have greatly lessened their hostility." Such historical examples may have found their way into the topical examination given each Byzantine envoy prior to departure on his embassy.[33]

As the handbook indicates, the Byzantines did not always live up to their reputation for generosity, especially in the last century of the empire, when scarcity of resources crimped both style and behavior. Calculation in making marital matches for diplomatic purposes was normally clothed in pomp and circumstance but, as we have already seen, the Byzantines hesitated and then fell to haggling over arrangements for Bertha of Sulzbach's marriage to Manuel I Comnenus, thereby threatening Byzantine relations with Germany at a critical time in the 1140s, when Byzantium needed German help against the Normans. A more stark example of the dangers involved in diplomatic stinginess is provided by the haggling that went on in 1195 A.D. between Muhyi al-Din, Emir of Ankara, and Emperor Alexius. The Emir hoped to take advantage of Byzantine willingness to buy off threatening neighbors but set his price too high for the emperor. Alexius III bargained and skirmished and departed for Byzantium, leaving a subordinate in the field. The emir laid siege to a Byzantine town and then defeated a relief army. The emperor settled for what was originally asked, but he did not get his city back.[34]

Another stark example in the empire's dismal last century of its departure from past generous custom was the altogether understandable but harsh and thus counterproductive treatment of 4,000 Norman soldiers captured in late 1185 and 1186 A.D. after they had ravaged the city of Thessalonica. Most were captured by a ruse, and numbers of them died each day for more than a year until, needing soldiers, the emperor released them into army service. Soon thereafter, they participated in a failed rebellion led by field commander Alexius Branas.[35]

The longevity of Byzantium can only be credited to its diplomacy and its generous strategy of pleasuring outsiders, which greatly mitigated but could not overcome or completely compensate for militarism, internal political divisions, religious fanaticism in both Rome and Constantinople, occasional maltreatment of resident foreign traders, and lack of resources. Nevertheless, Byzantium, by its intense diplomatic interaction over a millennium, with so many rulers, not only schooled the Christian and Muslim worlds in classical diplomacy and in the refinements that it developed over the centuries but also gave them a marvelous living example of the power of culture, beauty, pleasure, and money to defend a people and a way of life, and of the self-destructive nature of violence.

NOTES

    1. Walter Emil Kaegi, Jr., *Byzantine Military Unrest, 471–843: An Interpretation* (Amsterdam: Walter M. Hakkert, 1981), p. 27.
    2. Louis Brehier, *The Life and Death of Byzantium*, trans. Margaret Vaughan (Amsterdam: North-Holland, 1977), p. 21.

3. Ibid., p. 22.

4. Kaegi, *Byzantine Military Unrest, 471–843*, p. 11.

5. Charles Diehl, *Byzantium: Greatness and Decline*, trans. Naomi Walford (New Brunswick, N.J.: Rutgers University Press, 1957), pp. 7–11.

6. Brehier, *The Life and Death of Byzantium*, pp. 99–101.

7. Ibid., pp. 109–110.

8. Ibid., pp. 113–114.

9. Arnold Toynbee, *Constantine Porphyrogenitus and His World* (London: Oxford University Press, 1973), pp. 319–320.

10. Michael Angold, *The Byzantine Empire 1025–1204: A Political History* (London and New York: Longman, 1984), pp. 1–11. Arnold Toynbee observes that the annexation of Armenia during the years 1000 to 1045 A.D. was a fatal mistake by Basil II and his successors that would cost the empire Asia Minor. He likens it to the mistake Justinian I had made in 532 A.D. by liquidating "the Armenian princes and barons in the Roman Armenia of his day. The nemesis of the repetition of this error was proportionate to its geographical magnitude." See Toynbee, *Constantine Porphyrogenitus and His World*, p. 410.

11. Angold, *The Byzantine Empire 1025–1204*, pp. 24–25; Toynbee, *Constantine Porphyrogenitus and His World*, p. 345.

12. Angold, *The Byzantine Empire 1025–1204*, pp. 24–25.

13. Deno John Geanakoplos, *Byzantium: Church, Society, and Civilization Seen through Contemporary Eyes* (Chicago: University of Chicago Press, 1984), pp. 8–9.

14. Angold, *The Byzantine Empire 1025–1204*, pp. 110–111.

15. Ibid., p. 169.

16. Diehl, *Byzantium: Greatness and Decline*, p. 54. For the intelligence operations that fed this "science," see Francis Dvornik, *Origins of Intelligence Services: The Ancient Near East, Persia, Greece, Rome, Byzantium, the Arab Muslim Empires, the Mongol Empire, China, Muscovy* (New Brunswick, N.J.: Rutgers University Press, 1974), pp. 121–187.

17. Diehl, *Byzantium: Greatness and Decline*, p. 55.

18. Geanakoplos, *Byzantium*, pp. 202–203.

19. Rene Guerdan, *Byzantium: Its Triumphs and Tragedy*, trans. D.L.B. Hartley, with a preface by Charles Diehl (New York: G. P. Putnam's Sons, 1957), pp. 32–34.

20. Charles M. Brand, *Byzantium Confronts the West 1180–1204* (Cambridge, Mass.: Harvard University Press, 1968), pp. 20–23, reviews Byzantine marital diplomacy. See also Guerdan, *Byzantium: Its Triumphs and Tragedy*, p. 107.

21. H. W. Haussig, *A History of Byzantine Civilization*, trans. J. M. Hussey (New York: Praeger, 1971), pp. 189–190.

22. Guerdan, *Byzantium: Its Triumphs and Tragedy*, p. 19.

23. Haussig, *A History of Byzantine Civilization*, p. 191. The automata made such an impression on the Arabs that they developed even more sophisticated ver-

sions for their court in Baghdad. Indeed, the Arabs' reception of foreign envoys was perhaps even more magnificent than the Byzantines' and had of course the same purpose, to dazzle the envoys and convince them that the resources of the Arabic empire were inexhaustible. From refreshments of iced beverages and beer upon arrival to farewell gifts of hundreds of thousands of coins, Arab hospitality toward respectful envoys was unstinting. But whether more lavish or not in their hospitality, the Arabs strictly imitated the Byzantines' tight handling of foreign envoys. Byzantine and Arab control of diplomats was the model on which the much poorer Muscovite state based its own tight handling of diplomats. See Dvornik, *Origins of Intelligence Services*, pp. 251–254, 310–313.

24. Geanakoplos, *Byzantium*, pp. 22–23. Liudprand, the Bishop of Ancona, suffered a generally unpleasant reception when as an envoy of the German Emperor Otto II he sought a royal princess for the son of Otto. The Byzantines disdained the Germans and reacted harshly to the request. It was a miscalculation on their part and hurt them in the long run. See Guerdan, *Byzantium: Its Triumphs and Tragedy*, pp. 166–183.

25. Guerdan, *Byzantium: Its Triumphs and Tragedy*, p. 22; Haussig, *A History of Byzantine Civilization*, pp. 190–191; Toynbee, *Constantine Porphyrogenitus and His World*, pp. 505–506.

26. Angold, *The Byzantine Empire 1025–1204*, p. 166.

27. Geanakoplos, *Byzantium*, pp. 352–353.

28. Angold, *The Byzantine Empire 1025–1204*, p. 244.

29. Haussig, *A History of Byzantine Civilization*, pp. 195–196.

30. Guerdan, *Byzantium: Its Triumphs and Tragedy*, pp. 41–45.

31. Angold, *The Byzantine Empire 1025–1204*, pp. 159–163.

32. Ibid., p. 168.

33. George T. Dennis, trans., *Three Byzantine Military Treatises* (Washington, D.C.: Dumbarton Oaks Research Library and Collection, 1985), pp. 125–127.

34. Brand, *Byzantium Confronts the West 1180–1204*, pp. 135–136.

35. Ibid., pp. 160–175.

5

The Byzantine Doge and
the Parsimonious Prince

The supple diplomacy of Constantinople, with its eye on the present moment and its frequent recourse to the power of pleasure, was the model for
Western Europe. Through Venice, a longtime dependent of Constantinople,
and through direct contact, the ancient Roman diplomatic practices with
their Greek and Persian elements became the core of modern European
diplomatic practice. This style of diplomacy, with its strong emphasis on
the needs of the moment and the utility of pleasure, was expensive. Although recourse to pain and refusal to persevere in diplomacy ultimately
did Venice in, its use of pleasure and the strategic mobilization of its high
culture enabled the Byzantine protegé on the Adriatic to survive a millennium and more. Not surprisingly, the Venetian approach to international
relations produced a reaction on the part of states less willing or able to
mobilize wealth in this fashion. Their champion was Niccolò Machiavelli
of Florence, whose handbook, *The Prince*, was based on decades of diplomatic experience on behalf of the relatively small and much less wealthy
city-state of Florence. He counterposed Florentine parsimony and theory
to Venetian generosity and practical present-mindedness. Employing parsimony and pain to the virtual exclusion of pleasure kept Florence from
achieving Venice's grandeur. Venice, not Florence, became the model for
modern Europe.[1]

Both the domestic and foreign politics of Venice bore the mark of Byzantium. Venice survived its infancy as an independent state, because Constantinople protected it from Franks and Italians on the mainland. During
the three centuries before it betrayed Byzantium in 1204 A.D., Venice par-

asitized the Greek empire. In return for trading privileges, Venice offered
Constantinople naval services. In 1082 A.D., quite early in the unusually
long reign of Alexius I Comnenus, the parties formalized the relationship
in a treaty of alliance. From 1204 A.D., when it betrayed Byzantium, until
the fall of Constantinople, Venice had to reckon directly with the Ottoman
Turks, whom it alternately fought and parasitized. This unhappy duet
locked the partners into old ways that left them weakened in the face of
industrialized states. Finally, in 1797, Napoleon Bonaparte conquered Venice, and the City of Saint Mark lost its role as a diplomatic actor. The
Ottoman empire would last another century and a half, playing out its role
as "The Sick Man of Europe."

The origins of Venice as a cluster of a dozen desolate refuges from invading Lombards in the marshes and islets of coastal Venetia in 568 A.D.
were unpromising, but the people of these marshes and little islands won
Constantinople's favor. They helped both the Byzantine general, Belisarius,
against the Goths and another Byzantine commander, Narses, to move
troops in his Ravenna campaign. With the blessing of the latter, the islanders established their independence of Padua. In return for valuable
trading rights and privileges, they formally submitted to Constantinople.

In 697 A.D., the islanders unified under one leader, or doge, a title conferred by the emperor on the governors of the Byzantine provinces of Italy.
At the beginning of the ninth century A.D., Venice became a pawn in international politics as the Frankish and Byzantine empires struggled for
pride of place in European politics. In 809 A.D., under pressure from the
Franks, the islanders retreated to the middle of the lagoon, Rialto, the site
of modern-day Venice. In the following year, they came under attack from
Charlemagne's son, Pepin, and resisted strongly. Frustrated and sick, Pepin
was vulnerable. Operating well within Byzantine norms, the Venetians
bought him off. In doing so, they effectively bought their freedom, though
they were nominally Byzantine subjects, as a Franco-Byzantine Treaty of
814 A.D. confirmed. The Franks had sought Byzantine recognition of the
claim of Charlemagne to the title of Roman Emperor of the West. In this
treaty, however, the Byzantines only recognized Charlemagne as an emperor but did not legitimize his claim to joint rule of an empire tracing
back to Rome. Nonetheless, the Franks recognized Constantinople's theo-
retical hold over Venice.[2]

Caught between two empires, each of which refused to recognize the
claims of the other, the Venetians had to be both flexible and focused.[3]
Two decades later, they adopted Saint Mark as the patron of their republic.
By 840 A.D., Venice had negotiated its first written treaty known to history.

This document was formalized at Pavia and established a peace of five years' duration between Venice and the German empire, confirmed earlier trading rights and agreements, and defined trading areas for German and Venetian merchants. While they subsequently hosted in a magnificent fashion the German king's successor, they were careful to remain on good terms with both Germans and Byzantines. Indeed, Doge Orso I married the daughter of Emperor Basil I.

Venetian diplomacy, which was the model for Western Europe and eventually the rest of the world, followed the practices developed in Byzantium. Reliance on pleasure, or at least mutual advantage, was the hallmark of the Adriatic republic's ascendancy. Bribery was as important a diplomatic tool for Byzantium's little client as it was for the City on the Bosporus. Indeed, although bribery was a very common activity of European ambassadors in the Middle Ages, the Venetians were especially active in this regard. The Venetians studied their neighbors as closely as did the Byzantines for signs that bribery might be effective. For one set of negotiations with the king of Hungary, Venice armed its ambassadors with 5,000 ducats to spend on bribes for their Hungarian counterparts and 50,000 to 60,000 ducats to give to the king of Hungary. Later, after a review of the customs and conditions of the Hungarian nobility, the Venetian leaders gave Marco Dandalo, their ambassador to Hungary, 5,000 ducats to pass among the nobles and another 5,000 to bribe some key barons and the queen of Hungary herself.[4]

As a seagoing nation, Venice was concerned about suppressing piracy in the Adriatic and keeping any other nation from dominating that body of water. Policing was a more demanding chore than naval politics. Byzantium, its titular sovereign, had so let its navy decline that it posed no threat. In fact, Byzantium's weakness at sea provided the Venetians with an opportunity whenever Byzantine diplomacy could not ward off the City's seaborne enemies. Such was the case when the Anglo-Normans threatened Byzantium late in the eleventh century A.D. In May 1082 A.D., Venice and Constantinople entered into a treaty. Venice agreed to attack the Anglo-Normans and to continue to acknowledge the overlordship of Constantinople. In exchange, the Byzantines provided a title and an annual honorarium for the doge and his successors, twenty pounds of gold a year for the Church of Venice and an honorific title for its patriarch. They also granted the Venetians unrestricted trade free of customs duties throughout the Byzantine empire and port facilities in Constantinople and on the shore opposite Galata. This forever altered the economics of the empire and positioned Venice to become a major force in the eastern Mediterranean.[5]

The relationship between Venice and Byzantium was not always easy. Byzantine rulers were aware of the cost of Venetian trade privileges, and there was a recurring pressure to end them. Complicating matters still further, Byzantium never lost the longing to head a revived Roman empire. Pursuit of either goal upset Venice. Thus when Emperor John Comnenus sought to end Venetian trade privileges, the Venetian response was to attack the Byzantine islands in the Aegean and force John Comnenus to ratify all the Venetian trade privileges in a treaty of 1126.[6] Venice sometimes indulged Byzantine dreams of grandeur, sometimes not. In 1149 A.D., it joined a German-Byzantine alliance and helped Byzantium under Manuel I Comnenus retake Corfu from the predatory Norman king, Roger II. This triple alliance against the Normans and their allies, the Guelfs, France, Hungary, Serbia, and the Papacy, began the practice of widespread alliance building in Europe. These grand alliances precede by two and a half centuries the League of Venice against the invading French. Their fluidity was quickly illustrated when Emperor Manuel I subsequently failed in his attempt to wrest Southern Italy from the Normans and thereby alienated both Germany and Venice. Byzantium had overreached itself diplomatically and militarily and paid a heavy price for its dreams of military grandeur.[7]

The relationship of Venice to Byzantium deteriorated. The Byzantine alliance in 1169 A.D. with Genoa and in 1170 A.D. with Pisa, both rivals of Venice, further estranged the City from its protegé. Worse was to come. On March 12, 1171, the empire took a fateful step and had every Venetian in its boundaries arrested and his goods confiscated. Venice retaliated by attacking the Byzantine coast and sacking the islands of Lesbos and Chios. This resort to armed vengeance backfired. Not only did the violence fail to intimidate the Byzantines, but the fleet of the victorious doge, Vitale II Michiel, brought pest instead of plunder back to Venice from Byzantium. Distraught Venetians murdered their doge. It would be ten years before relations between the two states were restored and compensation made.[8]

But the Venetians sought more than compensation; they wanted revenge. And to that lust was added a desire for preeminence in the east. The result was a city-state turned empire, brought again and again to the point of extinction by its worst instincts and finally left to expire. First, Venice would have its revenge. The occasion for that revenge was the Fourth Crusade.

Long-lasting tension between Latin and Greek Christians, fed by the aggression of Constantinople in Italy and tactlessness toward the West by the Emperor Andronicus I, rankled Westerners and gave its more ambitious leaders an excuse to attack Constantinople under the guise of a crusade.

The Venetians were happy to offer transport, provided that the Crusaders helped them recapture the city of Zara, which had deserted to Christian Hungary. Having accomplished that, the Crusaders passed on to Constantinople, took the city in July 1203 A.D. and sacked it in April 1204 A.D. Venice joined in the partition of the empire and built one of its own. It took over three eighths of the City and a number of the important ports and islands in the eastern Mediterranean, including Crete. The Venetians had under their control the entire sea lane from Venice to Constantinople. It seemed a triumphant moment, a time when arms had triumphed over diplomacy and desperate defense.

For all the appearance of victory, Venice lost more than it gained. The fall of Constantinople to the Fourth Crusade meant that Venice no longer had an effective buffer between itself and its enemies to the east. That lack would have painful long-term consequences. Cooperation with the crusaders encouraged Venice to take part of Acre and part of Tyre, as well as many country estates near both cities. Venice thus exposed itself to loss and depredation in the turbulent Levant. Wrangling with Genoa over Acre led to war. Venice inflicted defeat after defeat on its Italian rival but, while its fleet was away from Constantinople, Michael VIII Paleologus seized Constantinople in 1261 A.D. and drove out the Venetians. Genoa, of course, backed Paleologus. In 1268 A.D., Paleologus allowed the Venetians to begin trading in the Byzantine empire, but they never again enjoyed commercial privileges as extensive as they had had before the Fourth Crusade.[9]

Overarching, militant ambition also flawed Venice's commercial policy, and with similarly painful results. Venice sought to force all traders doing business on the northern Adriatic to exchange merchandise at Venice. After about two generations, these irksome measures, which included a prior claim on food supplies in times of shortage, led to a war with resentful Ferrara. Venice lost. It had to pay a large indemnity, agree to supply the wheat Ferrara needed, and give up a canal project meant to undercut Ferrara's trade. But it kept its hold on shipping to Ferrara from the Adriatic.[10]

The reluctance of the Venetians to restrict their commercial rivalry with Genoa to measures short of war affected Venetian society in terribly crucial ways. Victories and defeats in the struggle for mastery of the Aegean and Black Sea and the straits between were equally dangerous and oppressive for the working-class citizens. They became more and more estranged from upper-class Venetians. Hard times further hardened class lines. The republic became more of an oligarchy. Meanwhile, members of the upper class fought among themselves to establish foreign policies that would favor their own families.[11]

After 1234 A.D., the Venetians abandoned their hope of restoring a Latin kingdom at Constantinople and became the protectors of the weak Byzantine state against both the Genoese and the Turks. The Black Death of the fourteenth century killed so many Venetians that it could no longer depend on its own citizens to man its navy. Nonetheless, in 1350 A.D., it plunged into war with Genoa and lost. Only a combination of clever Venetian diplomacy and Genoese civil unrest extricated Venice from its third war with Genoa. But within months of the conclusion of the war in 1355 A.D., King Louis of Hungary took advantage of Venice's debility by seizing nearby Dalmatia. Subsequent squabbling with Genoa over Cyprus led to loss of trade there. Then unrest in Cyprus led by local Venetians spurred the republic to dispatch a terribly expensive expedition of mercenaries which suppressed opposition to Venice's imperial rule. This sort of militant pursuit of commercial advantage left Venice with debased currency, a rising public debt, smaller trading opportunities, and a nagging tendency toward expensive protectionism.[12]

Within a quarter century, Venice was once more at war with Genoa. The Fourth Genoese War, "the War of Chioggia," was a disaster both for the victor, Genoa, and the defeated, Venice. The Venetians, relying heavily on mercenary troops, were barely able to defeat an attack on Venice itself. But clever diplomacy, including the willingness of Venice to buy support from the king of Hungary, and the exhaustion of Genoa saved the day for Venice. While the Treaty of Turin (1381 A.D.) was a masterpiece of diplomatic craft, it could not disguise the fact that pugnacity had cost Venice dearly.

Even after Venice's ill-fated descent from the slope of violent revenge against Byzantium and the pursuit of empires overseas and on the Italian peninsula, the bribe remained an economical, handy tool in the Venetian arsenal. When it came time to negotiate with the Turks, they gave their ambassador 500 ducats "to expend on those persons with whom he will have to treat for peace and other matters committed to the said ambassador." The Venetians also authorized their ambassador to buy gifts of silver and cloth for the Turkish chancellor and other courtiers. But these were modest allowances compared to that given in 1384 A.D. to the Venetian notary at the papal court whom the Venetians instructed to pay in cash and on the spot whatever it took to obtain the papacy's approval of trade with the sultan of Egypt.[13]

Within the Venetian nobility a faction was developing with an appetite for wealth drawn not from overseas but from the Italian mainland. With Venice bloodied at sea, desirous of secure trade routes across northern Italy and over the Alps, and dependent on raw materials from the mainland for her growing industry, those who called for expansion on the mainland received more attention. Over the quarter century down to 1406 A.D., Venice conquered more and more of the surrounding mainland. But the most ambitious expansionists had little patience for the intricate diplomacy necessary to deal with the other city-states in northern Italy: Milan and Florence. When the opportunity arose in 1423 A.D. to join Florence against an expansionist Milan, Venice chose to renounce peacetime prosperity for what turned out to be thirty years of ever more costly warfare in Lombardy. Eventually, all the political forces in Italy joined the contest on one side or the other, and sometimes on one side and then on the other.

War in peninsular Italy against the Milanese led to Venetian weakness overseas in the face of the expanding Turkish empire. The fall of Constantinople to the Turks was a shock to the exhausted Italians, who then agreed in the Treaty of Lodi (1454 A.D.) to make peace with one another and to wage war against the Turkish empire. All five major Italian powers—Venice, Naples, the Papal State, Florence, and Milan—agreed to join in a crusade, but Venice, which took a decade to enter the fray against the Turks, soon found itself almost alone. Despite initial military successes in Greece, and control of the sea in the final years of a sixteen-year-long war, Venice eventually lost. In January 1479 A.D., Venice signed a peace treaty which gave to the Turks some of her overseas possessions and 10,000 ducats per year for the privilege of trading in the Turkish empire.

While the public purse bore the costs of purchasing such common benefits, Venice expected its ambassadors to bear some of the financial burdens of diplomacy. As a result, ambassadorships to the more prestigious posts with their correspondingly high style of court life could be so expensive that even men of substantial wealth tried to duck the responsibility. They were all the more reluctant particularly if they could foresee difficulties in accomplishing their task.[14] As diplomacy became more intensive and embassies of longer duration, the problem compounded.

Generous abroad in their diplomatic pursuit of commercial opportunity, the Venetians were no less so at home when receiving foreign diplomats. The French ambassador, Philippe de Commines, remarked of Venice in his *Memoirs*, published in 1495 A.D., "It is the most triumphant city I have ever seen, does most honor to all ambassadors and strangers, and governs itself with the greatest wisdom."[15] While one might reasonably question de Commines' judgment on the political wisdom of the Venetians, he saw their diplomatic practice through seasoned eyes, and there is no doubt that the Venetians had carried on the Byzantine tradition of grand official hospitality. Inasmuch as it was still the custom at that time for receiving states to pay the costs of visiting ambassadors, the lines between gifts and bribes were sometimes murky.

The Venetians needed all the goodwill they could buy. In 1494 A.D., the French invaded Italy to take over Naples. Against the French, Venice organized a league which included the German emperor and the king of Spain. Spain was the new element for, of course, formal Venetian relations with the German emperor went back six and a half centuries. Though beaten on the field of battle, the League of Venice was successful, because the French king withdrew from Italy. Soon enough, Venice alienated its partners and found itself embroiled in war, with French support, for more Italian territory. The opportunistic Turks seized the opportunity to attack Venice's overseas possessions and to once more plunder their way nearly to within sight of Venice. Venice made peace in 1503 A.D. by yielding many cities in Albania and Greece. It retained little but just enough of the overseas empire, however, to tempt it into self-destructive policies in the centuries to come.

The Venetians of the early sixteenth century preferred to concentrate on building their Italian mainland empire. They thought that they could use a combination of mercenary armies and very clever diplomacy for that purpose. They underestimated, however, the opposition that their schemes would stir up and overestimated the strength of their mercenary forces. In December 1508 A.D., Pope Julius II rallied France, Spain, Austria, England, Ferrara, and Florence in the anti-Venetian League of Cambrai, still another great wartime alliance of sovereign powers. Its military forces having disastrously failed in battle and its mainland holdings gone, the Venetians pulled themselves together and struck back militarily and above all diplomatically. When the citizens of the liberated cities rose up against their cruel liberators, the Venetians took the field and regained a few cities. But mostly they relied on diplomatic skills to defeat the League. In the darkest hours of the war's first year, Venice bought off the king of Spain with the gift of ports in the Italian district of Apulia and attempted to buy off the pope and emperor as well.[16] Their ambassadors having publicly abased themselves in the presence of the Pope, the Venetians were soon allied with him against France, and the League of Cambrai was undone.

Initially effective in destroying the seemingly invincible League of Cambrai, the Venetian strategy of playing one power against another became obvious too soon. Eventually no gifts or ceremonies could completely smooth over the resentments and overcome foreign distrust of Venetian ambition. The result was a long, drawn-out series of wars lasting until 1529 A.D., when Venice adopted a successful policy of neutrality. Venice's wartime diplomacy was typically Veneto-Byzantine. Flawed as it was, Venetian diplomacy in this period was the shield of the republic and saved it from the ruin into which militarism would otherwise have plunged it.

Except for two wars in 1537–1540 and 1570–1573 A.D., fought in alliance with Spain and the Hapsburg monarchy against the Turks, Venice successfully maintained its policy of neutrality. The wars demonstrated clearly that peace was preferable to war. The first of the two wars cost Venice the last of its islands in the Aegean north of Crete. The second, despite the great naval victory over the Turks at Lepanto in October 1571 A.D., cost Venice its claim to Cyprus. The wars also illustrated the cost of the turn from sea to land. Even quintupling its fleet over the previous century and a half had not saved Venice. The wars in Italy as well as frequent outbreaks of plague and famine had taken their toll on Venice's strength. Furthermore, the preoccupation with land warfare had made its youth ignorant of the wider world of the seaborne merchant.[17] To blame the Venetians' slowness to go to war against the Turks on attachment to the pleasures of their city rather than on military overextension and natural disaster, as Cristoforo Da Canale, a naval expert, did in 1539, is wide of the mark.[18]

Pleasure indeed continued to serve the city well in its international relations. In 1574 A.D., the Venetians greeted the young King Henri III of France with splendor and pomp designed to make his stay a high point of his life. The goodwill and friendship of the French king were very important to the republic, so all of the citizenry participated in a welcome that rivaled the greatest Constantinople had given its most honored guests. The banquets and balls and the public entertainments were lavish. Privately, the great artist Tintoretto painted him, and Veronica Franco entertained him. He had chosen her from a picture book of the city's most beautiful courtesans. She wrote two sonnets in his honor.[19]

Venice's artists wandered Europe creating goodwill for the republic, and its courtesans were always entertaining. Nonetheless, at great and irrational cost, the republic persisted in clinging to the shreds of its old empire and pursuing self-destructive militarist ways. Venetian protectionism did not improve matters and indeed compromised Venice's position and prospects in international trade. Piracy only made matters worse and spurred the Venetians to dispatch a military expedition against pirates in the lands of the Austrian Hapsburg archduke. Diplomacy more than military conquest brought the affair to a successful conclusion in 1617 A.D. In 1628 A.D., Venice chose war again to meddle in the succession of rulers in Mantua, and Venetian diplomacy barely salvaged what had turned into a military debacle. Saddled with debt, the city then suffered another horrible visitation of the plague.[20] The Venetians held on stubbornly and at very great cost to Crete from 1644 A.D., when the Turks attacked it until its capital, Candia, fell in 1669, after a twenty-one year siege, the longest in Western history. Not only was there the cost of warfare to the people of Crete and Venice, but there was the loss of business to competitors from France, England and Holland. Such expenses and lost business were compounded by the disruption of the important German markets during the Thirty Years War of 1618 to 1648. For their part, the belligerent Turks weakened themselves enough that their subsequent ill-fated campaign into Central Europe was compromised and their defeat at Vienna in 1683 confirmed the perils of overextension.[21]

Venice's persistence in fighting for Crete impressed others as a sign of strength of character, all the more impressive coming from the pleasure-loving Venetians. But trouble would follow trouble, and some of it would just underline the folly of war. Another visitation of the plague followed two years after the loss of Crete. Venetian shipbuilding never recovered, though Venice's port activity grew through the end of the sixteenth century. Skilled manpower became expensive, technology stagnated, and more efficient and adventurous competitors with easier access to naval stores, such as the Dutch, flourished.

Persisting in expensive, self-destructive imperial pretensions like those that Byzantium had suffered, Venice went to war three times with the Turks between 1645 and 1718. It gained little of permanence, save some land in Dalmatia. In 1687, one of its gunners blew up the Parthenon in Athens during the temporary reconquest of Greece, a land soon lost again to the Turks. Venice was left with the considerable burden of a skyrocketing public debt. In contrast, her competitors, the rising powers of England, France, and Holland, fastened upon the weakening Turkish empire and gained for themselves lower tariffs of the sort that had once favored Venice in the latter days of Byzantium. Venice did not eliminate the advantage of her competitors until after peace with the Turks in 1718. Further compromising both the military strength and the diplomatic prowess of the republic was the reluctance of her nonartistic sons to travel abroad and learn the many ways of a changing world. The banter and badinage of salon society was no substitute for worldly experience.[22] The den had become too comfortable for the cubs of the Lion of Saint Mark.

There were some glimmers in this period of relative decline. Venice decided to pay tribute to the rulers of Barbary and profited mightily. When that strategy no longer proved effective, the Venetians went to war against the Bey of Tunis and vanquished his pirates' nest in 1784.[23] It likewise took advantage of its neutral status to rebuild its commerce during the American and French revolutions and the Russo-Turk wars of the eighteenth century. But the end was near. Led by nobles with too much to lose in a fight, it spurned a defensive alliance with other Italian states, abandoned even a pretense of diplomacy, and became a victim of Napoleon, who then looted it and made it a plaything of his imperial politics. Venetian unwillingness to engage in active diplomacy was a mortal error as the young Bonaparte could still have been thwarted by a determined Italian alliance. Fittingly, Napoleon had softened up the Venetians with bribes paid to the poorer members of the nobility.[24]

Southwest of Venice beyond the Papal States and Ferrara lay the city-state of Florence, which dominated the area of Tuscany in north-central Italy. Florence was not endowed with a favorable location, but its people were risk takers. Unfortunately, risk taking too often took the form of military adventures against neighbors and massive speculative loans to regal warriors. The drain of warfare and the reverses suffered by clients such as England's Edward III combined to end Florence's premier role in European finance.[25]

In 1513, Niccolò Machiavelli, citizen of Florence, wrote but did not publish *The Prince*, a booklet on governance that he finally dedicated to Lorenzo de' Medici. In that booklet, he distilled twenty years of diplomatic experience on behalf of his native city. The booklet's insistence that prowess, not goodness, is crucial for any ruler's success caused an uproar in Catholic Europe outside of France. "Any man who tries to be good all the time," argued Machiavelli, "is bound to come to ruin among the great number who are not good. Hence a prince who wants to keep his post must learn how not to be good, and use that knowledge, or refrain from using it, as necessity requires."[26] Machiavelli further opined that humans "are ungrateful, fickle, liars and deceivers, fearful of danger and greedy for gain" and consequently only fear, not love, could hold them in check.[27] A phalanx of moralists led by members and ex-members of the newly formed Society of Jesus, the Jesuits, responded that goodness was critical to success in governance.[28]

Doubtless, Machiavelli's failure to convince his fellow Florentines that alliance with the rising but unreliable French was shortsighted fed his mordant analysis of humankind. He also failed to convince in time the citizenry of his rich, geographically vulnerable republic that reliance on treacherous foreign mercenaries was no substitute for the self-reliance of a citizenry trained in military ways. By the time he had gotten a citizen militia organized, it was too late to harden them for a showdown with the battle-toughened Spanish, invited into Italy by the French. For their obtuseness, the normally alert Florentines paid with their freedom and fell under Medici control. Machiavelli was tortured as an anti-Medici plotter and retired to the countryside, out of active politics. Ever the teacher and presumably bored by his forced rustication, Machiavelli took on the task of enlightening the Medici about governance and international politics.

Machiavelli was leery of standing armies. He viewed them as more expensive than colonies and a source of inconvenience to everyone in the state. "Everyone," he argued, "feels this inconvenience, every man becomes an enemy; and these are enemies who can do harm, because even though beaten, they remain in their own homes. On every count, then, defense by armies is useless, as defense by colonies is useful."[29]

Not that Machiavelli was against the use of pain in international affairs. He simply preferred to use citizen soldiers whose mobilization was less expensive than that of mercenaries. For distant operations, he preferred colonies to armies, oblivious to the dangers of colonialism. To strengthen his point about the baleful effect of relying on mercenaries, he advanced the case of Venice. Venice, he observed, turned from a successful career as a sea power reliant on its own armed citizenry to a land power following the military customs of Italy, living in fear of its own mercenary captains, and then in 1509, at the battle of Vaila, losing its entire land empire in a single day.[30] To emphasize the point still more he brought up the case of the emperor of Constantinople, John V Cantacuzene, who, "in order to put down his neighbors, brought into Greece an army of ten thousand Turks; when the war was over, they refused to leave and thus began the enslavement of Greece by the infidels."[31] Clinching his case, Machiavelli argued that the basic reason for the fall of Rome was the hiring of foreigners, initially Goths.[32]

Gold had other limitations as far as Machiavelli was concerned. The Florentine argued that only exorbitant taxation or the distribution of war booty made generosity possible. The ruler's generosity thus rewards few but angers many and encourages them to long for a new ruler. The parsimonious ruler, by contrast, does not burden his people with taxes yet manages to defend himself against his enemies and undertake major works. In that age, it was the miser who accomplished great things; all of the others went under.[33]

Machiavelli's rejection of generosity was not complete. He grudgingly admitted its short-term utility in corrupting a regional lord who might open the way to an invasion of his liege lord's kingdom. While treachery might pave the way to victory, Machiavelli believed that other lords would rebel at the least opportunity and take over the kingdom for themselves.[34]

At least one other aspect of pleasure, flattery, was not altogether useless either. Indeed, flattery was a fearsome thing, a plague, and the prince had to be on guard against it. Only by giving wise courtiers a narrow license to tell the truth in response to specific questions could the prince protect himself from deceit.[35] Presumably, flattery would be useful as a diplomatic tool, but the Florentine did not explore that issue.

All in all, Machiavelli's *The Prince* is rather unsophisticated in its approach to statecraft, relying as it does on the pain principle and neglecting the pleasure principle in its discussion of international relations. While Machiavelli does encourage rulers to bestow prizes on those who open up a new branch of trade or in some special other way enrich the city or state, his basic assumption was that wealth was very hard to enlarge. Consequently, all members of society would suffer when wealth was sent abroad to bribe others. Thus can be explained his reluctance to endorse bribery of foreign officials. The perfidy of mercenary troops in the Italian peninsula strengthened his refusal to consider a more flexible diplomacy.

Machiavelli returned to his themes in a subsequent work, *Discourses on the First Ten Books of Titus Livius*. In it he pilloried the popular notion that gold was useful in diplomacy or war. After all, had not Solon said as much to Croesus, the fabulously rich king of the Lydians? Had not the King of Macedonia only drawn down the Gauls upon himself when he showed their envoys enough gold and silver, he thought, to frighten them? And had not the Venetians recently lost their entire state, while their treasury was still full of money? (Of course, here, as in *The Prince*, Machiavelli conveniently omitted the fact that Venice had survived and quickly regained all that it had lost.) "[G]ood soldiers, not gold, as common opinion proclaims, are the sinews of war," argued the Florentine, "for gold is not sufficient to find good soldiers but good soldiers are more than sufficient to find gold." Fearful neighbors of the steel-wielding Romans, for example, had been eager to give the Romans gold. Left conveniently undiscussed was the effectiveness of the gold in buying off the notoriously rapacious Romans, or for that matter the Romans' effective use of gold in buying off their enemies and in maintaining clients.[36]

Some of his Catholic critics in early modern Europe were less disingenuous than Machiavelli and certainly much more sophisticated. With the advantage of the perspective gained from the passage of time, they not only met Machiavelli on his ground of Roman history but they also drew from medieval European, Byzantine, and contemporary Chinese societies to demonstrate his limitations. They accepted the widespread practice of bribery; a few considered it essential. The Jesuit Netherlander Carlo Scribani wrote in *The Christian Politician*, published in Antwerp in 1624, that gold bought crucial intelligence about enemy states. "Nothing," he believed, "is impervious to gold, not even the marriage bed." The German Jesuit Adam Contzen, whose *Ten Books on Politics*, published at Mainz in 1621, was to become an important blueprint for statesmen in Central Europe for the next century, taught that it was better to win wars with money than with blood, a frequent anti-Machiavellian sentiment. The anti-Machiavellians were optimistic that economic development would produce the wealth needed for the state to pay the bribes without resorting to economic oppression. More fundamentally, they were optimistic that the good could survive and do well in politics.[37]

Bribery pervaded modern European politics. After studying centuries of archival materials, James Westfall Thompson and Saul K. Padover concluded that ambassadors had a threefold role: "lie, spy, bribe" and that "[t]he practice of bribing was a universally accepted diplomatic method. . . . A list of European bribes in this period would fill a good-sized volume."[38] In their eyes, Richelieu's tenure from 1624 to 1642 as France's champion in the field of foreign affairs was a triumph of words and gold. The cardinal's diplomacy led France to European preeminence and reduced Spain, for a century and a half the leader of Europe, to a third-rate power.[39]

Where gold was not accepted, expensive presents such as wine, horses, silverware, and pictures might be.[40] Early in the eighteenth century, France was diplomatically isolated and sought to entice England under the Hanoverian dynasty into an allliance. The Duke of Orleans, Regent of France during the minority of Louis XV, ordered an emissary to bribe King George I's Secretary of State, James, First Earl, Stanhope. Stanhope spurned a bribe of 600,000 livres. Undiscouraged, the French envoy, Abbé, later Cardinal, Dubois, sent to France for sixty cases of the finest wines, half for Stanhope and half for the king. The wine was enough to convince Stanhope. The king was unmoved; only the possibility that the alliance would protect his native Hanover finally brought him over. As French ambassador to London, Dubois, like Talleyrand later, "attached great importance to good dinners as means by which diplomacy might achieve its designs." His dinners featured all manner of French wines and delicacies. And, as Thompson and Padover note, he "was also a careful distributor of silks among his English lady friends. He knew precisely the effect an exquisite French taffeta would have upon the mind of a cabinet minister's wife. Dress designs, patterns, and weaves he studied as carefully as he did English politics."[41]

Dubois was careful in his cultivation of the English. He wrote to the Regent, "Nothing must be neglected in order to win the affection of the actors in this matter, both great and small; not by direct proposals, which might make them think that we believed them capable of being suborned, but by practice of such noble manners as will seem to partake rather of generosity than of design to ensnare their infidelity." Unfortunately for France, the Treaty of Hanover, as the alliance with England was called, turned out very badly because it led to the alienation of Russia and war with Spain, not to mention heavy subsidies for Sweden.[42]

An overview of Florentine history confirms the utility as well as the limitations of money in international relations. Machiavelli's Florence, capital of Tuscany, never enjoyed the stature of Venice. During his lifetime, it fell under the control of the Medici family. Rather than being parsimonious princes, the Medicis drained the city and province to support their vaulting political ambitions. They never developed the Tuscan economy enough to support a generous foreign policy without exploiting the Tuscans, but they did demonstrate the efficacy of money and sheer diplomatic effort in keeping alive a state. Careful to protect themselves and their Tuscan base of operations in the whirlwind of international strife, the Medicis sought neutrality at some cost to the city's prestige. Cosimo's purchase of Austrian support in the early eighteenth century was lavish enough to be hurtful to the Tuscans. Support from the Papal States was useful, but there was a high price to pay, hospitality to large numbers of religious congregations whose members had to to be supported and whose leadership had to be attended to. The hospitality was a heavy economic and political burden on Tuscany. Writing of the city's complex diplomatic history under the Medicis, J. R. Hale described the city as a "backwater" but noted that, "The absence of a major incident, which relegates Tuscany to a footnote in the history of international affairs, is a concealed tribute to assiduity rather than evidence of incompetence or indolence."[43]

NOTES

1. William J. Bouwsma, *Venice and the Defense of Republican Liberty: Renaissance Values in the Age of the Counter Reformation* (Berkeley: University of California Press, 1968), pp. 624–628. For the influence on the Venetians of "the Renaissance doctrine of the occasion, which was essentially concerned with the problem of action in a world dominated by forces beyond control," and the Venetian emphasis on history as a source of perspective rather than of lessons, see ibid., pp. 270–292.

2. Christopher Hibbert, *Venice: The Biography of a City* (New York: W. W. Norton & Co., 1989), p. 7.

3. George Ostrogorsky, *History of the Byzantine State*, rev. ed., trans. Joan Hussey, with a foreword by Peter Charanis (New Brunswick, N.J.: Rutgers University Press, 1969), p. 198, reviews the controversy surrounding this issue. I adopt his position that we are dealing here with a fruitless controversy about diplomatic formalities in which "[n]either the successors of Charles the Great nor the Byzantine Emperors ever obtained the confirmation of the other party."

4. Donald E. Queller, *The Office of Ambassador in the Middle Ages* (Princeton, N.J.: Princeton University Press, 1967), p. 94.

5. Ostrogorsky, *History of the Byzantine State*, pp. 358–359. H. W. Haussig, in the appendix to his *A History of Byzantine Civilization* (New York: Praeger, 1971), dates the end of the independent Byzantine economy by reason of privileges granted to the Italian city-states to the second half of the twelfth century. But he puts the beginning of the period of decline a half century later, when Byzantium was caught between the rising Ottoman state and the national states of Serbia, Bulgaria, and Hungary.

6. Ostrogorsky, *History of the Byzantine State*, p. 377.

7. Ibid., pp. 383–386.

8. Ibid., p. 389; Frederic C. Lane, *Venice: A Maritime Republic* (Baltimore: Johns Hopkins University Press, 1973), p. 35.

9. Lane, *Venice: A Maritime Republic*, pp. 75–76.

10. Ibid., pp. 65–66.

11. Ibid., p. 174.

12. Ibid., pp. 174–185.

13. Queller, *The Office of Ambassador in the Middle Ages*, pp. 21, 94–95.

14. Lane, *Venice: A Maritime Republic*, p. 324.

15. Ibid., p. 237.

16. Peter Lauritzen, *Venice: A Thousand Years of Culture and Civilization* (New York: Atheneum, 1978), pp. 125–126; Lane, *Venice: A Maritime Republic*, pp. 241–245.

17. Lane, *Venice: A Maritime Republic*, p. 248.

18. Hibbert, *Venice: The Biography of a City*, p. 96.

19. Ibid., pp. 100–101. Margaret F. Rosenthal suggests that Henri may also have met Veronica Franco through one or another of her powerful intimates. See Margaret F. Rosenthal, *The Honest Courtesan: Veronica Franco, Citizen and Writer in Sixteenth-Century Venice* (Chicago: University of Chicago Press, 1992), pp. 102–111.

20. Lane, *Venice: A Maritime Republic*, pp. 384–389, 400–402.

21. Lauritzen, *Venice*, pp. 174–175, 178–179. Hibbert, *Venice: The Biography of a City*, pp. 149–151, puts the siege of Candia (Iraklion) at twenty-two years.

22. Maurice Rowdon, *The Silver Age of Venice* (New York: Praeger, 1970), pp. 114–131, esp. p. 120.

23. Lane, *Venice: A Maritime Republic*, p. 419; Rowdon, *The Silver Age of Venice*, p. 131.

24. Rowdon, *The Silver Age of Venice*, p. 175.

25. Ferdinand Schevill, *History of Florence, from the Founding of the City through the Renaissance* (New York: Frederick Ungar, 1968), passim.

26. Niccolò Machiavelli, *The Prince*, trans. and ed. Robert M. Adams (New York: W. W. Norton & Co., 1977), p. 44.

27. Ibid., pp. 47–48.

28. Robert Birely, *The Counter-Reformation Prince: Anti-Machiavellianism or Catholic Statecraft in Early Modern Europe* (Chapel Hill: University of North Carolina Press, 1990), pp. 1–44, 217–242.

29. Machiavelli, *The Prince*, pp. 6–7.

30. Ibid., pp. 37–38.

31. Ibid., p. 39.

32. Ibid., p. 41.

33. Ibid., pp. 45–47.

34. Ibid., p. 13.

35. Ibid., pp. 67–68.

36. Niccolò Machiavelli, *The Portable Machiavelli*, trans. and ed. with a critical introduction by Peter Bondanella and Mark Musa (New York: Penguin Books, 1979), pp. 309–313, 191.

37. Birely, *The Counter-Reformation Prince*, pp. 136–138, 147, 163, 177.

38. James Westfall Thompson and Saul K. Padover, *Secret Diplomacy: Espionage and Cryptography, 1500–1815*, 2nd ed. (New York: Frederick Ungar, 1963), p. 58.

39. Ibid., pp. 77–78.

40. Ibid., pp. 112–113.

41. Ibid., pp. 120–122.

42. Ibid., pp. 123–124.

43. J. R. Hale, *Florence and the Medici: The Pattern of Control* (London: Thames and Hudson, 1977), pp. 183, 186, 190.

6

Lording It over the Britons:
England's Anglo-Norman Empire

While the Venetians were pursuing an empire and falling victim to their imperial ambitions, the descendants of the Norman conquerors of England built an overseas empire that ultimately would curse the island. Like Venice, Anglo-Norman England used a combination of force and pleasure to expand its influence and rule. Those whom the Anglo-Normans sought to conquer effectively used pleasure as a bulwark against Anglo-Norman expansion until the Anglo-Normans devised ways of overcoming it. Yet in overcoming pleasure, the Anglo-Normans ultimately diminished their own diplomatic tools and eroded the empire's strength.

After the Normans defeated the Anglo-Saxons in a closely contested battle at Hastings in 1066, they brought to England a new social order with pronounced characteristics. Norman society expected its leaders to prove their command of the wealth of society. They had to provide themselves, their courtiers, and their guests with wine, wheat bread, and venison killed by their own hands. So the Normans spent the first years of their consolidation of power in England trying to seize all of the wheat-growing land in England. They initially left the uplands, the oat and barley-growing areas, to the native Anglo-Saxons and Celts. Within a few generations, they had taken all of the lowlands and had moved into Wales, where they encountered fierce resistance and began to lose their foothold. Then the Norman-Welsh looked abroad for more wheat-growing land. Strife-torn Ireland, momentarily warm because of a climatic optimum that favored wheat growing, had the misfortune to be nearby. The Norman-Welsh readily answered an Irish lord's recruiters and involved themselves in Irish struggles after about 1166.[1]

With support from their Norman cousins in Wales, England, and France, the Norman-Welsh initially were successful invaders. In the lowlands of Hibernia, they defeated the Irish soldiers and systematically built castles and planted colonies of Welsh, English, and French agriculturalists. The upland Irish fought on in guerrilla fashion. The lowland Irish, however, turned to a pleasurable strategy of resistance that also drew on the deepest roots of their culture. Irish society was consciously and proudly different from that of the continentals and the Anglo-Saxons. For example, in medieval Ireland, as in Abyssinia at the other end of Christendom, Christianity "never seems to have really expanded outside the purely religious sphere of life . . . whereas in the remainder of Christendom, both Latin and Orthodox, it became a whole social system."[2] From as early as the Council of Whitby in 664 A.D., Irish Christianity resisted intense pressure from Rome to change. It refused to give up its Celtic ways or romanize the Irish people, especially its women. To the women, independent in their ways, fell the main defense of lowland Ireland after the Norman invasion. To them and their use of pleasure must go the credit for the ultimate failure of Norman rule in much of lowland Ireland. As lovers, wives, mothers, and foster mothers, they brought the Normans down.[3]

Irish women scorned continental women as mere pawns in financial and political bargaining. They treasured their own liberty to pick mates for the moment or for life.[4] They were choosy, preferring to lie with and marry males outstanding for their prowess in one field or another. Consequently, the Celtic males around them were highly competitive achievers with a proclivity for the singularly heroic. Having lost to the invading Normans, they temporarily yielded pride of place to the new champions whom Irish womenfolk would bed down.

By the mid-thirteenth century, "many of the principal Norman magnates were the grandsons of Irish twelfth century kings, and many Irish kings were the grandsons of twelfth century Normans."[5] Within two centuries the Normans beyond the Pale were the Irish-Normans and little Norman at that. In the eyes of Anglo-Norman cousins in Dublin with Anglo-Norman wives or across the Irish Sea intermarrying among the Norman cousins, they were more Irish than the Irish. For the victorious Normans, it was easy to adopt such local customs as the pursuit of champions by women.

David Beers Quinn believes that Irish influence over the Anglo-Normans grew from the thirteenth through the fifteenth centuries because the Irish

developed a professional soldiery. That soldiery was built around
hereditary soldiers, the "galloglass" (galloglaigh), and their families imported from Scotland. Faced with the threat of stiffened Irish resistance,
the English bought peace from the Irish by paying "black rents"—protection money.[6] Yet clearly the Irish women had many victories over the invaders. They seduced the Anglo-Norman overlords. Also, by extending the
Irish tradition of fosterage to the children of the invaders, they softened
the invaders and converted their children to Irish ways. It was common
practice in pre-Elizabethan Ireland for women of good social standing to
seek out the children of the ruling class to nurture them. The foster mothers
thus gained the protection and love of the parents whose children they
nursed and, in the eyes of one English observer, spoiled by extreme indulgence. The foster parents "nourish[ed] and hearten[ed] the boys in all vil-
lainy, and the girls in obscenity."[7]

In this same period, the foreign relations of England and France illustrated both the futility of power politics and the capacity of the pursuit of
pleasure, the sweetness of sugar, to sour international relations. Norman
ties encouraged England's rulers to meddle in the power politics of France.
The meddling drained much of England's military strength but produced
little in return. For their part, the French meddled in English court politics.
King Louis XI kept many people at the English court, including the English
king, on the French payroll.[8] One noteworthy development in the court life
of the thirteenth century or shortly thereafter was the habit of extravagant
marzipan displays at the noble table. The sugar for the confectionery displays came from the labor of unfortunate Slav captives put to work on
Mediterranean plantations—thus the name "slave" for captive laborers.
Demand for sugar increased as lower orders imitated the nobles. By the
sixteenth century, merchants were providing guests with marzipan displays.
Sugar became an important commodity in international trade; the wealth
produced by the slaves became a factor in international politics, and so did
places suitable for growing sugar, such as the Caribbean islands. England
and France especially had found something sweet to fight over for centuries.
The stakes became greater and the fight more bitter as sugar in one form
or another became a common stimulant and energy-packed food for the
emerging working class, whose womenfolk gave up the time- and energy-
consuming preparation of monotonous, traditional food and left their families to eat an inferior sugary diet.[9]

The search for profitable sources of sugar would be a motor in the rise
of England's overseas empire. The classical expression of the Anglo-
Norman theory of imperialism was *Utopia*, the work of Thomas More, a

successful, well-seasoned diplomat and lawyer. In that work, More describes the ideal foreign policy as one in which the core nation supplies unbribable, efficient administrators to neighboring countries upon request. Utopia makes no treaties, believing that treaties encourage hostilities between the parties involved. Utopia goes to war only in self-defense, to avenge a citizen whose death or disablement in a foreign land has deliberately gone unpunished, to repel invaders from the territory of allies, to help allies in redressing wrongs, or to liberate the victims of dictatorship. Taking the route of safety first, Utopians seek victory without battle by offering and always paying a huge reward for the heads of the enemy king and his associates, and twice as much to those bringing them in alive. The same amount and a pardon go to targeted officials who turn in others on the wanted list.

The Utopian bribe-first strategy usually works, according to More, because people will do anything for money, and the Utopians are prepared to pour limitless sums into its success. Where this approach does not work, the Utopians use a divide-and-conquer strategy first by bribing members of the enemy's ruling family or the leaders of countries surrounding the enemy state.

In this work and in his other behavior, More exhibited the great European Catholic culture and paid with his life for it. More's thinking on international relations has many parallels with the anti-Machiavellianism described in the previous chapter. More's advocacy of non-violent approaches to international relations also reflects the practical experience of Tudor England in its dealings with Ireland. Greatly weakened by the Black Plague, England under the Tudors sought to strengthen its hold over Ireland by offering titles to various Irish rulers and by gifts. Violent methods were of limited utility.

Under the Stuarts and the Puritan Commonwealth, pleasure would occasionally demonstrate its practicality in international relations, but violence became the favored instrument in English foreign policy. Diego Sarmiento de Acuna, Count of Gondomar, twice ambassador of Spain's Philip III to the court of James I, roused the hatred of Protestant Englishmen for the influence he developed over James. During his two terms as ambassador (1613–1618, 1620–1622), he developed a personal friendship with the English monarch based on several shared interests, particularly literature. He also kept the king and queen and several prominent English leaders on pensions. Using friendship and money, he kept England from intervening on behalf of Protestant factions in continental wars and drove the French ambassador from England.[10] While such forbearance irritated

English Protestants, it conserved English forces that could be invested in civil war and the subjugation of the Irish. The Irish suffered more than ever at the hands of the English. Victorious in England's civil warfare, the Puritans encouraged tens of thousands of Irish soldiers to leave the country and transported hundreds of thousands of Irish to Connaught, the bleak western part of the island.

Despite the deaths of hundreds of thousands of civilians and systematic attempts to destroy their culture, the Irish remained resilient. Most of the Puritan colonists found that they had to learn Irish, and their children became Irish speakers and often lost English completely. "This was," Peter Berresford Ellis reports, "even more pronounced among the ordinary soldiers of whom a great many married Irish women and were in a short space of time completely absorbed into the Irish nation." By 1697, an English writer observed that, "We cannot so much wonder at this [Irish cultural power of absorption] when we consider how many there are of the children of Oliver [Cromwell]'s soldiers in Ireland who cannot speak one word of English."[11]

Meanwhile, the French government set out to effect an Anglo-French alliance by exploiting the notorious venality, lust, and superstition of the restored Stuart court. King Louis XIV and his ambassador to England, Marquis Charles Colbert de Croissy, lured King Charles Stuart II with the prospect of a large trade with France that would throw off enough tax revenue to free Charles of dependence on Parliament. Leaving nothing to chance, they bribed King Charles II's venal mistress, Barbara Villiers, Lady Castlemaine, and scattered gifts among the other women of the court. They also sent an Italian priest with a reputation as an astrologer. Instructed to interpret omens in a way favoring the proposed alliance, the priest failed miserably when Charles immediately put his powers to the test at a local racetrack. Money and sex were more reliable political tools; the French Foreign Ministry quickly dispatched jewels to Lady Castlemaine—"and jewels always go down well with ladies, whatever their mood," wrote the Foreign Minister. Having forged the French alliance in the secret Treaty of Dover (1670), Charles requested as a parting gift from Louis XIV Louise de Kerouaille, handmaiden to his beloved sister Henriette Anne, Duchess of Orleans. Upon repeated requests, Louis XIV dispatched Louise de Kerouaille with instructions to seduce Charles II and strengthen his ties to France. The coy Frenchwoman did as she was told.[12]

The English of course were not above trying to bribe foreign officials. Money and presents to a minister's family, with or without a foreign monarch's knowledge and acquiescence, were meant to sway a foreign government. Sometimes the bribe might be more imaginative. Historian Peter Barber reports that "British envoys in Stockholm in the 1720s offered education at Eton to leading ministers' sons."[13]

The sugar bonanza and the corruption of the English body politic would taper off in the 1720s but not before England had embarked on a crusade to overwhelm and destroy Scotland as a potential ally of France, the great competitor for sugar. The Act of Union of 1707 united the kingdoms of England and Scotland in a new kingdom, Great Britain. Many lowland Scots, particularly those of Glasgow, were eager and able to take advantage of the broadened trade opportunities, much as the Greeks had been of the Persian empire two millennia before. Nevertheless, until nearly 1750, the economy of Scotland as a whole languished. There was such discontent that in 1715, 1719, and again in 1745–1746, Highland Scots sought to overthrow the reigning Hanoverian dynasts and restore the Stuarts to the throne of England.

The English finally stamped out the rebellion with a combination of ruthless force against the rebels and, eventually, generous patronage toward their allies. Much as they had done in Ireland, they destroyed local political, social, and cultural patterns, including language and costume. Scots leaders were hanged, transported to penal colonies, or driven into exile. Historian Lawrence Henry Gipson wrote that, "Despite the eventual restoration of the forfeited estates and the return from abroad of exiled leaders, the population suffered indescribable miseries in the course of the changing economic order."[14] Forty-five Scots were admitted into the House of Commons. Many others found employment as soldiers or junior officers in the British army or navy, useful tools in foreign wars where they could be little threat to the imperial homeland. Still others received diplomatic posts. As historian Peter Barber noted, "[D]iplomatic posts were a means by which Scotsmen could be given office and eventual award, and the Scots as a whole conciliated, without unduly offending English susceptibilities—out of sight, out of mind. As a result, in 1770, Scotsmen represented George III in Vienna (Stormont), Prussia (Mitchell), Russia (Cathcart), Poland (Keith), Naples (Hamilton), and Brussels (Gordon)."[15] To support the Scots and the Anglo-Irish on the government payroll, England spread the burden of its domestic and imperial needs for patronage onto the shoulders of colonial subjects in Ireland, the Caribbean, India, and North America.

The extension of English power, and therefore patronage opportunities, in the Indian subcontinent was all the easier because it was facing a much decayed Mughal empire. The Muslim Mughals had exploited the subcontinent, diverting its resources from production to devastation. What they did not spend on warfare and administration, especially tax collection, they spent on, in the words of Rhoads Murphey, "monument building and gorgeous display in an effort to legitimize power."[16] Repeated English efforts to gain favorable conditions in Mughal India for their merchants failed until 1715. Then the coincidence of Mughal decay and generous and self-abasing English diplomacy produced two years later concessions that were to become the basis for English expansion and power in the subcontinent. The presents offered to the emperor and the money scattered to the crowds of Delhi bore great fruit over time.[17]

To pacify the East India Company, the Mughal emperor had granted it an exemption from all transit taxes on imported goods and those purchased for export. But the Mughals did not clearly limit their concession, and their carelessness brought them much trouble. Company officials not only exercised this corporate exemption to build the fortunes of the company, but they also took advantage of it in their own private business activities. Then their appetites whetted by the profits arising from this edge over their local competition, they began to hire out their certificates of tax exemption to frustrated competitors. Over time, this financially weakened the Mughals but yielded individual Englishmen great wealth. Those who survived the grueling change of climate retired to England as wealthy young men whose arrival overshadowed old money and threw into confusion established elites.

From fortified bases in Madras, Calcutta, and Bombay, the English watched the disintegration of Mughal power and protected themselves against anti-foreign Indians such as the Nawab of Bengal. When he retaliated against the English for strengthening their fortifications at Calcutta, they engaged and defeated his forces in battle at Plassey in 1757. Clive, the victorious English leader at Plassey, may have owed his victory over the larger Bengali forces to the bribery of key Bengali units by Indian merchants. They preferred the prospect of peace and security under English rule to the chaotic uncertainties of Indian rule.[18]

With their windfalls, imperial subjects returning from India could flaunt great wealth, buy seats in Parliament, and exert considerable influence. Despite inoculation against such disruptive behavior by the earlier excesses of the Caribbean sugar planters, the English body politic reacted with intense fear and jealousy. Envious moralists objected to the old Elizabethan buccaneering spirit that possessed the East India Company's employees in Bengal.[19] Yet for all the outrage over the scale of the new wealth, the desire for wealth and patronage never slackened. In its ongoing wars with France, British leadership now sought to maximize the number of overseas positions available to its scions and to minimize the costs of maintaining such a network. French interests in the Caribbean were attractive, and French activities in India needed to be checked if East India Company posts and revenue were to be maintained. But the Caribbean and India were pest holes. North America, less physically dangerous than India or the Caribbean, the source of more modest windfalls and the market for the emerging English manufacturing sector, became ever more attractive.

In its quest for more numerous patronage opportunities and greater national wealth, the English leadership took the path of war with France for control of India and North America. In the competition with France for influence over the pieces of the splintered Mughal empire, the British used their superior financial resources to good advantage against the French, who were led by the Comte de Lally, son of an Irish Jacobite, in the dual post of governor-general of all the French establishments in India and commander-in-chief. Lally's fierce hatred of the English, courage, and competence could not compensate for his arrogance, tactlessness, impetuosity, and impecuniousness. Ultimately he and his troops were defeated and captured at Pondicherry on January 16, 1761, by English forces led by Anglo-Irishman Sir Eyre Coote.[20]

Rapacity sometimes carried everything before it. The relations of the English with Mir Kasim, Nawab of Bengal, demonstrate the limitations of warm diplomatic ritual, the peril of withdrawing generous privileges and, ultimately, the limitations of generosity. The corruption of the Englishmen in Bengal had riddled the finances of Bengal for decades and imperiled relations between the East India Company and the Nawabs. In 1762, Mir Kasim, recently installed as Nawab of Bengal, decided to bring the issue to a head. He had tried and found wanting the normal methods of diplomacy and gestures of hospitality and friendship in his dealings with the Company's representative, Sir Eyre Coote: "In every respect, I have done everything to please and satisfy him, and entered into mutual engagements with him; notwithstanding which behaviour, he has not consented to a single thing I have requested of him." Since the English refused to end their private abuse of the Company's customs duty exemption, Mir Kasim abolished all customs duties throughout his territories, thus depriving the English of their unfair advantage. The English went to war, defeated Mir Kasim, and replaced him with another Nawab. This prompted James Mill to write of the episode in *The History of British India*, "The conduct of the Company's servants, upon this occasion, furnishes one of the most remarkable instances upon record, of the power of interest to extinguish all sense of justice, and even of shame."[21]

Still, the English never forgot the power of money. Using subsidies to attract support from continental Europeans and North American colonials alike, England won the Seven Years War (1756–1763). There was, however, a sour, violent side to England's treatment of its North American colonies that was a foretaste of what was to come after victory. The English navy pressed hundreds of North American sailors into deadly involuntary servitude on its warships.

The size of the postwar public debt terrified English leaders and made them even more reluctant to provide peacetime subsidies to would-be allies. Prewar suspicion that peacetime subsidies were worthless turned into a guiding principle. When the Russian court at St. Petersburg sought both an annual subsidy and an alliance against the Ottoman empire, it ran up against this newly hardened English parsimony. The English government's parsimony alienated the Russians. Adding to the speed with which the nations were drifting apart was an episode of personal promiscuity on the part of Sir George Macartney, English Envoy in St. Petersburg, 1764–1767. Macartney seduced and impregnated one of Catherine II's ladies-in-waiting, who was also a cousin of the Russian foreign minister. Annoyed at the breach of etiquette, Catherine II banished the woman from the court, and the foreign minister made clear that Russia would not accept the reappointment of Macartney to a diplomatic post at St. Petersburg.[22]

Much of the debate over the structure of the empire that followed the successful conclusion of the Seven Years War with France focused on the problem of reducing the public debt while still securing enough reasonably safe but lucrative employment opportunities for the offspring of England's Anglo-Norman rulers and those of their English, Scot, and Anglo-Irish allies. Ireland was safe enough but used up as a source of lucrative employment or emolument. India was dangerous, and the payouts so lucrative that they were socially and politically disruptive—about twenty persons who had served in India were in 1768 members of Parliament. Under the rotten borough system, the purchase of parliamentary seats was possible for commoners of great means, and the newly rich returnees from India had comparatively great means, even though the East India Company and the people of Bengal did not seem to prosper.[23] North America, in contrast to Ireland and India, was safe and provided generous but not disruptively large patronage opportunities.

The need of the British empire for taxes and patronage to extend to those from the home islands was something that was obvious to contemporary American observers such as John Lendrum, Timothy Pitkin, and Mercy Warren. Pitkin tied the shift to the desire of George III and indeed all

English mercantile society to batten upon the American colonies and monopolize the wealth thereof. Pitkin compared the English to misers. Quite reasonably, the North Americans wishing to preserve their liberties resisted extension of the English patronage system.

English voices calling on the government to offer patronage to Americans were rare. The government paid them no heed. In 1765, a prominent English physician called on his compatriots to "promote scholarships for Americans in our universities; give posts and benefits in America to such Americans as have studied here, preferably to others." Dr. John Fothergill argued, "If the Government permit such youth to come to Europe on account of their studies, to come over in the King's ships *gratis*, we shall still unite them more firmly." He argued that hosting Americans in English universities would increase English interest in America and would "cement friendships on both sides, which will be of more lasting benefit to both countries, than all the armies that Britain can send thither."[24] The need for patronage was no less on the mind of the English governor of Massachusetts, who had been in office during the Stamp Act Crisis of 1765. He felt sorely the lack of patronage to build a local following and complained in 1768 to an English lord, "If Punishments & Rewards are the two Hinges of Government, this Government [Massachusetts Bay] is off its Hinges; for it can neither punish nor reward."[25]

The English oligarchy cast about for politically inexpensive ways of increasing taxes while still finding opportunities for themselves and their merchant and industrial allies. The result was a decade of trial and error that ended in war and the loss of most of their North American colonies.[26] One act which frustrated elites in North America, who were land speculators, and many frontierspeople, too, was the Proclamation of 1763. This law closed off the West beyond the crest of the Appalachians and preserved it for the Indians, the British and Scottish merchants who served them, and British placeholders. Another act, the Quebec Act of 1774, allowed the Catholic Church freedom in conquered Quebec and extended that province south to the Ohio River to block further expansion by English speakers. Together these two laws presumably lessened the need for a large military establishment to pacify French Canadians and Indians. To support the military needed to clear the frontier and provide patronage opportunities, taxes were to be exacted from the colonies and a quartering act passed to provide for local, immediate military needs. The Sugar Act of 1764 created more opportunities for traders in Britain while restricting the trade of North Americans. The Townshend Acts were meant to keep North American industry from competing successfully with nascent British industry.

Finally, the tea tax was to protect the East India Company, source of much government and elite income and patronage.

The colonials bitterly resented their degradation from the ranks of Englishmen to British subjects. As British subjects they would be subject to taxation without representation. They would not be allowed in victory to treat French Canadians as the English had treated the Irish and Scots. They could expect to be taxed at the will of Parliament, overwhelmed by troops, and made to support an established and a hateful church as well as innumerable placeholders, many of them absentees. Their industry and agriculture would be subject to discrimination in favor of English firms. Their shipping could be restricted and even eliminated. In short, they would be treated as the Normans had treated the Anglo-Saxons and as Anglo-Normans had treated the Irish and Scots and as they themselves, when enjoying English status, had treated aboriginals in eastern North America.

The situation of the colonials would have been worse but for the pleasuring activities of their agents in London. These agents were usually members of Parliament or close associates. They lessened the impact of the Sugar Act of 1764 and helped in the repeal of the Stamp Act in 1766. Historian Lawrence S. Kaplan explained that their success in these and other matters "was no mystery. Theirs was not really an arcane art. Private parties and discreet dinners had always been mutually pleasant paths to the confidence of the important middle echelon in the ministries, the more or less permanent secretaries and undersecretaries who bore the brunt of the responsibility for carrying out as well as presenting cabinet programs."[27]

In the decade after the French and Indian War, the English oligarchy created relatively few posts funded by taxes not under the control of the colonial legislatures. Still, the oligarchs managed to convince the colonials that they would create as many as they could. They moved relatively few troops into North America, but in 1768, when they rushed troops to Boston from Ireland to put down opposition to the imperial regulations, they nourished colonial fears of an Irish fate. Moving the settlement line westward in 1768 failed to erase the parallels with army behavior in Ireland and Scotland that had emerged when English troops burnt down frontier farms beyond the Appalachians. Plans to increase army forces in North America and to restrict trade and industry and westward expansion increased colonial dread.

In the early 1770s several tens of thousands of alienated lowland Scots, Ulster Scots ("Scotch Irish"), and Northern British borderers who shared a warrior ethic and distinct Celtic-influenced British culture joined the long, growing stream of Irish emigrants to America. All these enemies of the

Crown tipped the balance against loyalty to England.[28] Many of those from England had made their home in Ireland with English government support and at the expense of Irish speakers. But outrageously greedy English land-lords, most notably the Marquis of Donegal, drove them and the Irish Catholics from their homes and made them even more bitterly anti-English. They were eager to take a stand against England.

Colonial English Americans, who had made their homes and fortunes at the expense of aboriginals, Africans, and indentured Irish and Scots, had only to look upon the people from Ireland and the Scottish borderlands to see their own future as Britons. They rebelled. The Irish and, to a lesser extent, the "Scotch-Irish," eagerly joined them in a bitter war. The mother of rebel leader Patrick Henry described the war as "another set of 'lowland troubles.' "[29] General Thomas Gage wrote from North America to Lord Dartmouth on September 20, 1775, "Emigrants from Ireland have arrived also at Philadelphia, where we are informed Arms were immediately put in their hands upon their landing. There are many Irish in the Rebel Army, particularly amongst the Rifle-Men."[30] So prominent were the Irish in the coming of the war and its conduct that Johann Hinrichs, a Hessian mer-cenary officer hired by England, described it as "an Irish-Scotch Presbyte-rian Rebellion."[31] The rebellion also found great favor with the large German population. German-speaking Americans equated the English threat to property with a threat to liberty and flocked to the rebel cause.[32]

The war between England and its North American colonies was long and, by European standards, especially post-Napoleonic European stan-dards, a protracted guerrilla war characterized by skirmishing.[33] As was its custom, England contracted with German states for soldiers, the most fa-mous of which came from Hessen-Kassel. Thus it would be able to keep its own men "employed at home in manufactures and farming, while other armies bled themselves on the battlefield."[34] Overall, England employed more than 30,000 Germans, known to history collectively as Hessians.[35] The German mercenaries made up a third of the English forces in 1778 and 37 percent of the English forces in 1781. Apart from their scouts, the Jaegher, and light-armed grenadiers who were regularly in combat, the slow-moving Germans functioned as garrison troops and rarely fought. Garrison duty was boring and dangerous. Of the 19,000 soldiers from Hessen-Kassel, nearly 5,000 died, 90 percent from disease and exposure.[36] Consequently, they became increasingly vulnerable to a seduction strategy aimed at them from the outset of the war by rebel leaders and informally expanded by North American women.[37]

The American Congress offered foreign deserters from the English army who chose American citizenship fifty acres of land. Rebel handbills appeared among the Germans offering private soldiers fifty acres and non-commissioned officers and officers up to a thousand acres; in January 1778, livestock was added to the offer. Conditions permitting, the rebels treated German captives well, showed them the wealth of the countryside, and returned them to their units in the hope that they would lure away their fellows. When they kept the captives and put them to work, the Germans were usually well treated and well paid. Many began living with American women. Only when the Americans won enough victories to demonstrate that they might win the war did the troops from Hessen-Kassel begin to desert. During the English retreat from Philadelphia in 1778, 236 Hessians deserted; this figure equals 44 percent of the 535 Hessians killed in battle by the Americans during the whole war.[38]

With each subsequent American victory, the lure of free land and live-stock became more powerful. Congress offered the Germans everything needed to set up a farm, except a Hausfrau, but, as Atwood points out, "American girls soon made up for this discrepancy, beginning in winter quarters in 1777–78." Even more important than the desire for land and a new life in encouraging the Germans to desert, Atwood tells us, "were the attachments which Hessian soldiers formed with local girls and their families whenever they were in garrison or captivity. On closer examination the colonists found the bloodthirsty Hessians not so fierce after all. The Hessians for their part thought American women very attractive. References to their good looks, fine hair styles, and clean clothes, as well as to the predominant role they played in American life, are legion in Hessian journals." The Americans were wonderful hosts. Their custom of "bundling" in bed unmarried male visitors with unmarried daughters happily surprised the Germans and speeded the process of getting acquainted. The Germans understood that if passion led to impregnation, they would have to marry the daughter or support her and their child. Up and down the Atlantic coast, American women lured away Germans and others from the British armies. The women of Savannah were noteworthy for their activity in this regard.[39]

Pleasure in bed, at the board, and in the dance hall did not win the American Revolution but it did distract the English leadership, keep them in the cities, and offset some of the power of their money to buy auxiliaries and use them against the colonials. The offer of free land and livestock was also a powerful incentive. By war's end, 3,014 of the 18,970 Hessians who constituted two-thirds of the German mercenaries mustered into English service, and the most reliable had deserted to the American side.[40] That is more than five times as many as the Americans had killed. While the annual desertion rate may have been lower than in contemporary European campaigns, it must be remembered that desertion to the side of strangers in a strange and distant land is more difficult than desertion close to home.

The English army in North America did not have a chance to win as long as it was unable to live continuously and spartanly in the field. It was like the Roman army in Spain rotting in pleasurable cities, while the countryside successfully resisted halfhearted inroads. In 1777, General Burgoyne plunged south dragging a baggage train of comforts into the New York forests in a poorly coordinated campaign. He suffered disaster at the Battle of Saratoga. Ninety percent of the Americans' arms and ammunition at that battle had come from vengeful France.

Encouraging the French to provide more aid and to enter a formal alliance with the North American colonies was the fascinating, titillating, and ultimately successful Benjamin Franklin, who represented the Americans in France.[41] The colonials' choice of the shrewd septuagenarian as their diplomat was inspired. Franklin, the Philadelphia entrepreneur, inventor, practical philosopher, publisher, and publicity hound, was one of the most famous and prestigious individuals in Europe and America. He provided the American cause a lustre and leverage far beyond what a group of rebel colonies would normally have had in monarchical circles, and he skillfully played upon the French desire to avenge their loss to England in 1763.

The contrasting failure of English diplomats to effect a reconciliation with the colonies in 1778 is instructive. They were not authorized to placate the colonists in any substantial way. They were unable to recognize colonial independence or to abandon imperial claims to control trade, commerce, and patronage. The imperial ruling elite could not bring itself to reinvent the English political structure. It merely repeated its mistakes. In 1781, the English General Cornwallis led his softened troops from the comforts of port cities into the southern hinterland without support from the navy. He lost his army to a Franco-American force at Yorktown. The English cause went from disaster to disaster, weakened by pleasure and crippled by poor strategy. With their cause clearly unwinnable, the English sought terms of peace by sending an old friend, Richard Oswald, to sound out Franklin about a separate peace. The pleasure of friendship softened the old Philadelphian, and he hinted at a separate peace, apart from the French and in violation of the Franco-American alliance. Generous terms quickly induced the Americans to make peace, for they too were incapable of winning the war by force of arms.

From the rebels' side, the major factors in their victory were the love of liberty, the seductiveness of the women revolutionaries, the desire of old enemies for revenge on the English, and the ability to muster through diplomatic means the financial and political support needed to outlast the English. Enough men and women conspired and acted through means sweet and sour to oppose the imposition of English law and martial might. In both the cities and the countryside, colonial women sweetly demoralized the enemy. In the countryside, colonial men mauled the softened armies that ventured out from the cities. Using French military supplies, Irish and Ulster Scot emigrants and transported English convicts serving in regular army and militia ranks inflicted terrible losses on English troops. Joseph Galloway, former Speaker of the House of Assembly of Pennsylvania, testified to a House of Commons committee that about one-half of the rebel army was composed of Irish, one-quarter of English and Scots, and only one-quarter of natives of America. In 1778, General Sir Henry Clinton wrote from New York to Lord George Germain, the Secretary of War, that "The Emigrants from Ireland were in general to be looked upon as our most serious antagonists." At sea, Irish sailors such as Commodore John Barry, who founded the U.S. Navy, took such a heavy toll of English shipping that in his diary Governor Thomas Hutchinson misidentified Scotsman Paul Jones as Irish. When the war was over and the English beaten, Parliament member Luke Gardiner told his fellows that, "I am assured, from the best authority, the major part of the American army was composed of Irish, and that the Irish language was as commonly spoken in the American ranks as English. I am also informed that it was their valour determined the contest so that England had America detached from her by force of Irish emigrants."[42] And, of course, the fractious Irish kept English troops pinned down in Ireland, so great was the English fear that the rebellion might spread from North America to Ireland. Finally, and not least importantly, America's diplomats, chief among them Franklin of Philadelphia, and its Delaware Valley merchants maintained the colonies' credibility and credit even when the rebels had shown themselves unable to win a decisive military victory. As a result, vengeful France, a reluctant Spain, and the Netherlands contributed war supplies. France eventually sent troops and ships against the faltering English.

England's predatory foreign policy had failed terribly. England lost much of its empire. Yet the failure might have been worse. Against a broad historical backdrop, England was fortunate that the North American colonials were so localistic and that the strength of the British navy protected En-

gland from a full-blown attempt by rebellious colonials to seize power in
the heartland in the manner of rebellious Roman, Chinese, Spanish, or
Portuguese frontier forces.

It is not surprising that, after the Americans won their freedom from
England, they moved to abolish primogeniture, entail, and government establishment of religion. As those legal devices of the feudal state were torn
down in state after state, the institutional supports needed to sustain the
Anglo-Norman order in the thirteen newly freed colonies collapsed.

During the War for American Independence, the British aristocracy did
begin to clean up the rotten borough system, but its patronage problem
grew ever more challenging. India was forced to assume more and more of
the burden. Warren Hastings, as governor-general of Bengal, had to subordinate to considerations of political patronage his drive to fill posts in
Bengal with men of real merit. In 1781, he wrote to the directors of the
Company to explain that the English colonial government in Bengal really
needed few civilian officials but had 252. He explained that, " 'Many of
them [were] the sons of the first families in the kingdom of Great Britain,
and everyone [was] aspiring to the rapid acquisition of lakhs [of rupees],
and to return to pass the prime of their lives at home.' " Historian Penderel
Moon comments that "The process had begun whereby, in Mill's words,
India provided 'a vast system of outdoor relief for Britain's upper classes.' "[43]

Having lost America by grasping so strongly for its patronage opportunities, the British political establishment nonetheless tightened its control
over the East India Company and removed Warren Hastings as governor-
general. Henceforth, with just two exceptions, British aristocrats would
lead British operations in India. The dimensions of the patronage problem
can be grasped from a speech in Parliament by Dundas, a friend of Pitt,
longtime president of the Board of Control established by Parliament to
control the Company and himself a patron of a flock of fellow Scots in
India. Dundas unabashedly urged the appointment of Lord Cornwallis as
governor-general: "Here there was no broken fortune to be mended! Here
was no avarice to be gratified! Here was no beggarly, mushroom kindred
to be provided for! No crew of hungry followers, gaping to be gorged!"
But in his first stint as governor-general, rather than reducing posts available to Britons, Lord Cornwallis intensified the anglicization of British rule
in India. This policy led to the exclusion of Indians from all the higher
posts of Company administration in India and a growing separation between Indians and Westerners.[44] Through scarce-bridled greed, the English
elite and their Scottish confederates undermined English rule in India. En-

gland was repeating in India the very mistake that had alienated most of its North American colonies. Only the vast size of India put off the inevitable Indian reaction.

From the French Revolution of 1789 until the defeat of Napoleonic France in 1815, the Anglo-Normans spent most of their time trying to maintain a dominant position in European affairs and hold their empire together. To harm the French economy, they seized American ships trading with the French West Indies. To check the Americans, they held on to the frontier forts promised in the 1783 peace treaty and incited American Indians against the American frontier people. They even built a fort on acknowledged American territory. The angry Americans responded with a hurtful embargo on all foreign trade and sent John Jay to London to wring concessions from England. He was met with wine, feasts, flattery, and concessions meant to tie America to England as a most favored trading partner. England abandoned its forts in the Old Northwest and its Indian allies too, but it would not abandon its claimed right to impress American seamen or open its West Indies ports to large American trading vessels or important American staple crops. Jay wrote to President Washington of the flattery and the personal attention of Lord Grenville, England's negotiator, "So far as personal attentions to the envoy may be regarded as symptoms of goodwill to his country, the prospect is favorable. These symptoms, however, are never decisive; they justify expectation, but not reliance." Thus clear-eyed and fortified against English negotiating tactics but hampered by American weakness, Jay abandoned the traditional American claim that "free ships" meant "free goods" and submitted to arbitration of claims against American debtors. He also included in the treaty an article permitting English subjects with land in America to hold it and pass it on to their heirs on the same basis as American citizens. This was frightening, because Grenville's family had extensive claims to land in North Carolina. Americans took little comfort from reciprocal rights in England.[45]

Given the possibility of war with the Americans, there was a sharper edge to the perennial English fear that Ireland would be an ally and a staging ground for their continental enemies, so English statesmen deployed the full range of craft and might to choke off that possibility. To control the Irish Parliament, the English used the patronage list. To lead the Irish away from the traditional, seductive cultural patterns and into a more regulated, sexually repressed way of life in which Irish women would be less likely to try to seduce English forces, England called upon the Roman Catholic Church. England gradually restored the civil rights of Irish Catholics. Under the leadership of the brilliant William Pitt in the 1790s, the English government sponsored the establishment and operation of a seminary for the training of Roman Catholic priests at Maynooth. It also allowed European trained, and especially French trained, Roman Catholic clergy to enter Ireland. Many of them were steeped in Jansenism, the Roman Catholic equivalent of Calvinism, and after the outbreak of the French Revolution, with monarchism and anti-republicanism, values of a more immediate utility to the English government.

Inducing cultural change was an inspired, long-term strategy. In the short term, terror was the main English instrument, whether to crush urban riots or uprisings by Protestant and Catholic tenants. When the example of the French Revolution encouraged Irish Presbyterians to believe that Catholics too had it in their hearts to seek liberty and Anglican reformers joined Irish Catholics, Ireland seemed to be moving in the direction of a republic. But John Fitzgibbon, lord chancellor of Ireland and Earl of Clare,"led the government to suppress what it could not corrupt. . . . He was Irish born and Irish bred but Fitzgibbon did not think like an Irishman. He did not even think British; he thought English." Under his direction, the English government attempted to suppress Irish republicanism. His successor followed the same path and waged a bloody, merciless war in Ireland in response to the Rising of 1798. That war set the tone for the next two centuries of government violence and violent resistance to government in Ireland.[46] It is of more than passing interest and relevance to the question of the origins of the War of 1812 between England and the United States that one of the punishments visited upon more than a thousand Irish Catholics suspected of being members of a Catholic self-defense organization was involuntary servitude in the English navy, a harsh fate and harsher still on men who were almost all farmers and not seamen.[47]

In the following two centuries, the Irish suffered terribly but took advantage of English weakness after World War I to achieve partial freedom from England. Where once the sexual wiles of the Irish women had confounded Puritanism, they seem to have failed in the eighteenth through twentieth centuries. Was it merely, as Ellis believes, that "Time for assimilation was something that Ireland did not have?"[48] Or were other factors weakening the Irish ability to assimilate the English, factors other than the traditional divisiveness which the English exploited? Certainly the English systematically destroyed the economic and political bases of the Irish high culture. When the Irish population surged after the introduction of the potato, the old channels of cultural transmission could no longer reach the whole population. That population, moreover, was so miserably poor that it could not afford to learn or sustain much of the culture, much as the Roman peasantry could not learn or participate in the Mediterranean Hellenic culture. Having decapitated Irish society, in the late eighteenth century the English leadership adopted a new strategy of altering the sexual mores of the Irish women who might otherwise seduce the occupiers as they had the Puritans. In religious matters, as noted above, England switched from a policy of persecution of Roman Catholicism to one of co-option. It allowed European-trained, and especially French-trained, clergy to enter Ireland and reform the Irish Catholic Church along continental and Calvinist lines, weakening Irish culture and turning the tide against sex and its anti-foreign uses in Irish culture. The generosity of the English leadership toward Roman Catholicism in the late eighteenth century was slow in coming but remarkably effective in damping down the sexuality of the Irish, especially the women.

In 1803 the British, under Governor General Wellesley and General Lake, who had recently crushed the Irish Uprising of 1798, decided to crush the remaining Indian polity, the Mahratta Confederation. They set out to weaken their enemies before attacking them in the field. The British and Anglo-Indian mercenary officers in the Confederation army were an important but discontented element, because they were poorly paid and their extensive responsibilities were never recognized with a promotion to rank above captain. So when Wellesley offered to guarantee their pensions if they left the Confederation armies, a majority of the "good, regimental fighting officers" came over to the British and left gaping holes in the command structure of the armies opposing Lake. Suspicion unraveled the structure still more. Perron, a Confederation general of French background, dismissed all of his British officers; some Indian generals executed British officers who hesitated to fight against their countrymen. And the common soldiers drew the conclusion that all of their foreign officers were about to betray them. The result was an overall weakening of Mahratta resistance and the hastening of the Confederacy's demise.[49]

England's dealings with the United States during the Napoleonic wars demonstrated ham-handedness rather than cleverness. Problems with getting enough seamen for the English navy and merchant marine led to impressment of American seaman, a cause of war with the United States. The shortage of men also led to a growing number of unmarried English females, an increasing number of whom became active in the foreign missions, especially in the Middle East and India (after 1813). That would lead to the problems described in the next chapter.

NOTES

1. William E. Kapelle, *The Norman Conquest of the North: The Region and Its Transformation, 1000–1135* (Chapel Hill: University of North Carolina Press, 1979), pp. 213–230, esp. pp. 219–220; Liam de Paor, *The Peoples of Ireland: From Prehistory to Modern Times* (London: Hutchinson; Notre Dame, Ind.: University of Notre Dame Press, 1986), pp. 94–96, 102–103.

2. Kenneth Nichols, *Gaelic and Gaelicized Ireland in the Middle Ages* (Dublin: Gill and MacMillan, 1972), p. 3.

3. Ibid., pp. 16–18, 79.

4. For a general discussion of the sexual freedom of Ireland in this period, see ibid., pp. 73–77.

5. de Paor, *The Peoples of Ireland*, p. 103.

6. David Beers Quinn, *The Elizabethans and the Irish* (Ithaca, N.Y.: Cornell University Press, 1966), pp. 2, 15–16.

7. Ibid., p. 84.

8. Donald E. Queller, *The Office of Ambassador in the Middle Ages* (Princeton, N.J.: Princeton University Press, 1967), p. 94.

9. Sidney W. Mintz, *Sweetness and Power: The Place of Sugar in Modern History* (New York: Viking, 1985), pp. 13–15, 88–97, 118–119, 128–131, 146–147, 152–155, 182–186.

10. Peter Barber, *Diplomacy: The World of the Honest Spy* (London: The British Library, 1979), p. 67.

11. Peter Berresford Ellis, *Hell or Connaught! The Cromwellian Colonization of Ireland 1652–1660* (New York: St. Martin's Press, 1975), pp. 110–111, 248–249.

12. Allen Andrews, *The Royal Whore: Barbara Villiers, Countess of Castlemaine* (Philadelphia: Chilton Book Co., 1970), pp. 186–210.

13. Barber, *Diplomacy*, p. 103.

14. Lawrence Henry Gipson, *The British Isles and the American Colonies: Great Britain and Ireland 1748–1754* (New York: Alfred A. Knopf, 1966), pp. 179, 155–184. It is not surprising that Gipson, the first Rhodes Scholar from Idaho and an ardent Anglophile, found English atrocities "indescribable." Left undescribed, they cannot disturb public perceptions of the benevolent advance of empire and cannot inform or challenge historians such as Linda Colley, whose *Britons: Forging the Nation 1707–1837* (New Haven, Conn. and London: Yale University Press, 1992) inaccurately portrays the process of unification as essentially more seductive than violent and destructive (see pp. 119–132).

15. Barber, *Diplomacy*, p. 69.

16. Rhoads Murphey, *The Outsiders: The Western Experience in India and China* (Ann Arbor: University of Michigan Press, 1977), p. 52.

17. Ibid., pp. 56–57.

18. Ibid., pp. 57–59.

19. Penderel Moon, *The British Conquest and Dominion of India* (London: Duckworth, 1989), p. 7.

20. Ibid., pp. 64–70, 76–80.

21. Ibid., pp. 95–100.

22. H. M. Scott, *British Foreign Policy in the Age of the American Revolution* (Oxford: Clarendon Press, 1990), pp. 108–112.

23. Moon, *The British Conquest and Dominion of India*, pp. 289–290, notes the grievous disappointment of Arthur Wellesley, whose victory in 1800 over the Mysoreans established British paramountcy in India but whose reward was "only" an Irish marquisate and an annuity worth 5,000 pounds sterling. "I will confess openly," he wrote of the marquisate, "that as I was confident there had been nothing Irish or pinchbeck in my conduct or its results, I felt an equal confidence that I should find nothing Irish or pinchbeck in my reward." On the envy and suspicion stirred up by the returning "nabobs," see pp. 143–147.

24. Richard W. Van Alstyne, *Empire and Independence: The International History of the American Revolution* (New York: John Wiley & Sons, 1965), p. 28.

25. John Phillip Reid, *In a Defiant Stance: The Conditions of Law in Massachusetts Bay, the Irish Comparison, and the Coming of the American Revolution* (University Park: Pennsylvania State University Press, 1977), pp. 144–145.

26. Robert W. Tucker and David C. Hendrickson, *The Fall of the First British Empire: Origins of the War of American Independence* (Baltimore and London: Johns Hopkins University Press, 1982), pp. 213–316, prefer to view the period of the Stamp Act and Townshend Act crises as one of appeasement by Great Britain toward the colonies. In their view, "Appeasement is nearly always marked by self-deception. To believe that it is undertaken for reasons other than fear and a sense of impotence is part of its pathology. For the appeaser, the will to believe is substituted for the will to act" (p. 231). Such a judgment is inexplicable coming as it does hard upon the authors' evidence that the British leadership and they themselves considered a war against the Americans to enforce a measure, the Stamp Act, economically ruinous to both parties (p. 230).

27. Lawrence S. Kaplan, *Colonies into Nation: American Diplomacy, 1763–1801* (New York: Macmillan, 1972), pp. 22–23.

28. For figures on this emigration, see David Hackett Fischer, *Albion's Seed: Four British Folkways in America* (New York: Oxford University Press, 1989), pp. 608–610. I believe Fischer does not account adequately for the Irish.

29. Ibid., p. 779.

30. Reid, *In a Defiant Stance*, p. 209, n. 16.

31. Rodney Atwood, *The Hessians: Mercenaries from Hessen-Kassel in the American Revolution* (Cambridge: Cambridge University Press, 1980), p. 160. Atwood terms Hinrichs' view "completely ludicrous" and traces it to Hinrichs' poor comprehension of spoken English. He takes the indefensible position that coming from a completely different political and social system, the Hessians could not have

understood anything about the politics of the war (ibid., pp. 162–165). Hinrichs' terminology is more accurate than the common term "Scotch Irish." The Irish were far more active in the war against England than the Scots who tended to favor the empire which had by that time begun to reward it with patronage. Scots and borderers were numerically secondary to the Irish in this rebellion. Henry Jones Ford, who argues that "the sense of political communion between Ireland and America was very close," follows the English historian Lecky in the judgment that "the ejected tenants of Lord Donegal formed a large part of the revolutionary armies which severed the New World from the British Crown." See Henry Jones Ford, *The Scotch-Irish in America* (Princeton, N.J.: Princeton University Press, 1915; reprint, Hamden, Conn.: Archon Books, 1966), pp. 458–491.

32. A. G. Roeber, *Palatines, Liberty, and Property: German Lutherans in Colonial British America* (Baltimore: Johns Hopkins University Press, 1993), pp. 304–310.

33. Atwood, *The Hessians*, p. 235.

34. Ibid., p. 32.

35. Ibid., p. 157.

36. Ibid., p. 238.

37. Ibid., p. 186.

38. Ibid., pp. 186–188, 193, 196, 255–256.

39. Ibid., pp. 192–198.

40. Ibid., p. 256.

41. Thomas G. Paterson, J. Gary Clifford, and Kenneth J. Hagan, *American Foreign Relations: A History to 1920*, 4th ed. (Lexington, Mass.: D. C. Heath and Co., 1995), pp. 12–14.

42. Michael J. O'Brien, *A Hidden Phase of American History: Ireland's Part in America's Struggle for Liberty* (n.p., 1919; reprint, Freeport, N.Y.: Books for Libraries Press, 1971), pp. 74–97, 109–110, 159–161. O'Brien's analysis is that about three of eight rebel soldiers were Irish (ibid., pp. 134–135).

43. Moon, *The British Conquest and Dominion of India*, pp. 216–217.

44. Ibid., pp. 223–231. Ronald Hyam, *Empire and Sexuality: The British Experience* (Manchester, England: Manchester University Press; New York: St. Martin's Press, 1990), pp. 116–117, errs by attributing Cornwallis' actions to fear of an Indian uprising, similar to that which took place in Haiti after 1791.

45. Jerald A. Combs, *The Jay Treaty: Political Battleground of the Founding Fathers* (Berkeley: University of California Press, 1970), pp. 151–152.

46. Reid, *In a Defiant Stance*, pp. 135–159, esp. pp. 144–145, 154–155.

47. Ibid., p. 140.

48. Ellis, *Hell or Connaught!*, p. 249.

49. Shelford Bidwell, *Swords for Hire: European Mercenaries in Eighteenth-Century India* (London: John Murray, 1971), pp. 219–220.

7

The British Empire:
Doomed in the Fleshpots of Paris

The war against Napoleonic France lasted from 1793 to 1815. Following traditional patterns of international behavior, Britain poured millions of pounds sterling into foreign aid, building up and encouraging the continental neighbors of France to struggle together against the French empire. For the period 1793–1816, the total of all subsidies and loans amounted to only 8 percent of the expenditures on the army, navy, and ordinance. Subsidy payments tended to run at about 14 percent of the government's growing revenues. British leaders found it much more profitable to sweat and grind up their compatriots in mine and mill than to send them to murder or be murdered on the continent. Guineas, as the British coins were known, gunpowder, and other war supplies, along with strenuous coalition building, were critical ingredients in the victory.[1]

The high point of Britain's coalition-building efforts was the Treaty of Chaumont, signed on March 9, 1814, which laid out guidelines for the conduct of the war against Napoleon. The treaty also established an automatic mechanism for the post-war preservation of the balance of power among the great powers of Europe for at least twenty years. It was explicitly aimed at any French attempts to take revenge on any of the signatory powers. The pact also contained broad language committing the signatories to put "an end to the miseries of Europe," and to secure "its future repose, by re-establishing a just balance of Power, and ... maintaining against every attempt the order of things which shall have been the happy consequence of their efforts."[2]

While the coalition powers were formalizing their relationships at Chaumont, their plenipotentiaries were negotiating with the French plenipotentiary and foreign minister, Caulaincourt, at Chatillon, a deserted village on the upper Seine. Caulaincourt tried strenuously and cleverly to preserve for France at least some of the territorial gains made by Napoleon's armies. From February 7 to March 19, the diplomatists negotiated. Caulaincourt did his best to see to the envoys' pleasure, in the spirit of Francois de Callieres' century-old handbook on diplomacy, *On the Manner of Negotiating with Princes*. De Callieres had encouraged French diplomats to employ banquets for diplomatic ends and reminded them that "It is well known that the power of feminine charm often extends to cover the weightiest resolutions of state. The greatest events have sometimes followed the toss of a fan or the nod of a head." Caulaincourt brought out bounteous shipments of the choicest French viands and epicurean wine to all the ministers. A British participant remembered "that the conviviality and harmony that reigned between the ministers made the society and intercourse at Chatillon most agreeable. . . . [N]or was female society wanting to complete the charm, and banish ennui from the Chatillon congress, which I am sure will be long recollected with sensations of pleasure by all the plenipotentiaries there engaged."[3]

French hospitality was in vain. Too little and too late, pleasure did not save the bloodstained Napoleon. He abdicated and went into exile in April. The warring powers signed the Treaty of Paris on May 30, 1814.

To celebrate and to work out their hopes for the future, Europe's nobility and England's leaders flocked to Vienna for a Great Congress in September 1814. Emperor Franz II played host. Nearly bankrupt a few years before, he laid out 30 to 40 million gulden to make things pleasant. Hosting five emperors and kings, eleven ruling princes, ninety plenipotentiaries, and fifty-three non-invited representatives of European powers was a tremendous enterprise. The balls and mutual pleasuring were extravagant by any standards. Beethoven produced new music for the occasion.

Austrians groaned under a 50 percent tax increase meant to pay some of the costs and suffered from inflated currency. A university official worried that students and faculty members were demoralized and that the library was unable to buy books. There was grumbling but no revolt. The spectacle was entertaining, the gossip titillating. The government threw open many events to the populace and, following local custom, government and notables shared the food from the bounteous tables with the poor. Moreover, locals jacked up rents and prices to take what advantage they could of the visitors.[4]

The diplomatic stakes were very high, so diplomacy was not left to the diplomats alone. Nor was the diplomacy by any means all formal. The major players had extensive armed forces and numerous political officials at their disposal. They had learned that carnage was terribly expensive, even with British subsidies, and also that diplomats would probably not resolve the difficulties by themselves. In calculated fashion the principals, therefore, brought other techniques to bear. Diplomacy functioned everywhere, in ballroom and bedroom, bringing Austrian Prince de Ligne to remark that, "The Congress dances but it does not march." Was Austria's Metternich, the Congress's major diplomatic figure, a womanizer? Well then, the Russians would deploy his former lover, Princess Catherine Bagration. Bagration was a petite, exquisitely beautiful, charming little blonde lady, a distant relative and a great favorite of the czar himself, who had borne Metternich an illegitimate daughter after an affair in 1802. Bagration, whose budding love affair with the czar caused a tremendous stir in Vienna, was just one of "those diplomatic sybils whose mission," Countess Ludovica Thurheim reported, "was to gain friends abroad for Russia's political aims. Metternich," she added, "was [Catherine Bagration's] favorite lover, but others also ([Metternich's secretary] Gentz, for example) found a sympathetic ear with the lusty Russian lady. The familiar epithet applied in diplomatic circles to the princess was 'the beautiful nude angel' because of the deep décolleté she was in the habit of wearing."[5]

However much calculation was involved in all the erotic interplay, there is no doubt that passion finally took the monarchs in its grip. On a side trip with Emperor Franz to Budapest, Czar Alexander I was heard to whisper with some frustration and anticipation to Countess Orczy, "I am sorry not to have an opportunity for being conscience-struck but I hope to see you again in Vienna." After reading the memoirs of numerous participants and excerpted secret police reports, one author remarked of the Congress that it was the historical acme of women's international political influence, solidarity, and "communality of aims and methods of attaining them, a communality that embraced all castes, classes, and families, so that in the end there remained but little difference between empress and cocotte, and even the best of circles took no umbrage when the Danish king, half in fun, half seriously, permitted his low-class mistress to call herself 'queen.' "[6]

Francois de Callieres would not have been surprised by the influence of the women who attended the Congress of Vienna. Nor would he have been surprised at their ability to pry state secrets from the diplomats. He had warned the diplomats to be wary of love. The diplomat "must never forget that Love's companions are Indiscretion and Imprudence, and that the moment he becomes pledged to the whim of a favoured woman, now matter how wise he may be, he runs a grave risk of being no longer master of his own secrets." While he believed that "terrible results follow[ed] from this kind of weakness," it is hard to see any negative consequences of eroticism at the Congress.[7] On the contrary, it served to divert the monstrous egos of the aristocrats from their normal mischief and ensured that there were few if any political surprises.

Slowly, very slowly—no rulers wanted to rush back to their dreary courts and ordinary routine—the framework for a century of general European peace went up. Of secrecy, there was little or none. The hosts had spies everywhere, and most of the boudoirs oozed information. Still, the interests of and the conflicts between the various parties were fairly obvious; the difficulty lay in accommodating the former while minimizing the latter. So while the leaders indulged themselves and enjoyed one another's company, their minions worked out the details of agreements. Contemporaries tended to see the extravagance, not the work of diplomacy.[8]

Frivolous it may have seemed, but when the Congress ended on June 9, 1815, the ardent players had won, and the weak and clumsy had lost. Czarist Russia went away with a large portion of Poland and substantial diplomatic strength. From September through November 1815, it forged ties with Austria and Prussia that Europe knew as the "Holy Alliance," a reactionary combination against the democratic and nationalistic currents of the day. Austria used the Congress to extend its hold on north and central Italy and to bury the Hapsburg feud with the Bourbons that had plagued Europe for centuries. Prussia grew stronger. France, aided by deep divisions among its enemies and the adroit diplomacy of its Foreign Minister, Talleyrand, survived the Congress with minimal territorial loss and hobbled by an indemnity it would later reduce. France, however, had lost so many men in the Napoleonic wars that it was set on a downward path from the first rank of nations. The secondary states at Vienna did not mount an effective diplomacy nor did the hangers-on at Vienna, the princelings dislodged by Napoleon, none of whom had the resources to impress and win over the leading diplomats. The secondary states received scraps at best or were carved up themselves. Many of the princelings never regained their principalities. And, sadly, the republics of Genoa and Venice were formally absorbed by Piedmont and Austria, respectively, without the approval of their inhabitants, victims of the prevailing reaction and their own weakness.

The British were clumsy in the diplomatic game and thus less fortunate than the other major actors. With their money, they had made it possible for the continental Allies to win a war. But with the arrival of peace, English stinginess and desire to maintain a foreign policy based on military strength reasserted itself with the usual consequences. Long cut off from the habits of the continental rich, they appeared asocial and out of place at Vienna. One observer claimed that English "national pride prevents adaptation to others. Caught in a faux pas, they claim this to be the custom at home. On leave, they spend the day sightseeing in the city and its environs. In the evening they visit the few families that will receive them. Then they talk with ladies of easy virtue and get drunk on Hungarian wine." Public drunkenness marked the Englishmen, a "coarse, hippy walk," the Englishwomen. Castlereagh, the Irish landlord, and his wife were seen as parsimonious window shoppers in a city where the jewels on ball gowns were worth millions of francs. At least one English agent, Fortbrune, did make himself attractive enough to become one of Princess Bagration's lovers, but he could extract no information from her.[9] For all their hard drinking and wenching, the English diplomats at the Congress of Vienna escaped the fate of British plenipotentiary Charles Whitworth, whose death in 1725 has been attributed at least in part to participation in the overeating and festivities that marked the Congress of Cambrai (1724–1725).[10]

More important to the limitations on Britain's success at Vienna than the social gracelessness of its diplomats was its continued reliance on a militarized foreign policy. Unable to imagine national security without British supremacy on the seas, Britain's rulers and diplomats did no more than push for a balance of power scheme for Europe rather than a general reduction in armaments. Long fixated on the threat from across the Channel, they fostered a strong Prussia to balance the potential power of France. In the twentieth century, their descendants would die by the hundreds of thousands as a result of their failure to press for disarmament. So, while the Concert brought a temporary peace to Europe, it squandered the opportunity to achieve a more enduring peace. Ironically, one gain that Britain did salvage from the Congress, limitations on the Portuguese slave trade, was purchased with concessions in money and colonies, not extorted by threat of force. Further demonstrating the power of gold, Britain in 1817 bought Spain's agreement to abolish the slave trade. It is also of interest that when the vicomte de Chateaubriand took the post of French ambassador in London in 1821, he employed as embassy chef the renowned Montmirel, remembered for creating beefsteak Chateaubriand and pudding a la Chateaubriand (afterwards Pudding Diplomatic). Chateuabriand intended that "The French embassy, so long forgotten in this country, should once more take a leading place in pleasures as in affairs. The influence of society extends to politics, and where diplomacy is concerned, balls are by no means useless to the king's service, but that part of my job is not the one I like best."[11] Chateaubriand's aloof personality undercut the utility of pleasure and he was unable to warm the cool English elite. In the generally peaceful decades that followed, pleasure would find itself increasingly discounted and force increasingly valued.

The imprudence of cultivating military mechanisms to redress political and social problems in Europe soon manifested itself to Britain's leadership. The militarized, static European system born at Chaumont and celebrated at Vienna quickly came up against the nationalistic and liberal trends of the day. Armed defense of the status quo led to foreign intervention and repression of political discontent in Italy and Spain. The British made clear their position on non-interference with the internal affairs of other nations in a memorandum on the treaties of 1814 and 1815 submitted by their plenipotentiaries at the Conference of Aix-La-Chapelle in October 1818.[12] The prospect of European intervention in recurrently tumultuous Ireland alarmed the British government and drove it out of the European system. As George Canning, Britain's Secretary of State for Foreign Affairs, noted in a memorandum of December 12, 1824, he had found in French newspaper accounts of Ireland an "expression which is identical with that employed by the French Government to justify the Invasion & Conquest, & now the retention of Spain. Naples—Piedmont—Spain—Ireland!—who shall draw the line, if the principle of 'European question' be once admitted?"[13] The subjugation of Ireland haunted England's leaders and weakened their country.

As a conservative power now committed to non-intervention, England focused its diplomatic energies on the maintenance of British commercial opportunities throughout the world and on suppressing the slave trade. It also sought to sharpen the competitiveness of its diplomats and consuls by forbidding them, from 1834, to accept gifts from any foreign government, "an abandonment of one of the oldest diplomatic traditions."[14] But to smooth relations with one of its oft-annoying competitors, the United States, it resorted to bribery. England, through the Baring banking concern, kept on retainer Daniel Webster, a prominent politician who became the American secretary of state. The policy paid off; the notoriously greedy Webster represented the United States during negotiations over the border between Maine and Canada. The resulting Webster-Ashburton Treaty of 1842 ceded much of the land claimed by the United States to England and drew fire from many Americans. It also removed much of the friction from relations with America and can be considered a minor triumph of English gold.

The bribery of Daniel Webster was as smooth as things got in English diplomacy. The clumsiness noted at the Conference of Vienna occasionally reasserted itself. English dealings with Seyyid Said, sultan of Muscat and Zanzibar, are illustrative. In 1834, the sultan offered a 74-gun warship to the Royal Navy only to have his offer refused by a British government wary that acceptance might imply unconditional support for the sultan. The sultan then had the ship sailed to London where, after some delay, the English government accepted it, reciprocating with one of the king's finest yachts and membership in the Royal Geographical Society. The sultan refused the yacht on the grounds that a good Muslim might only pray in an unadorned setting and so gave the yacht to the governor general of India, who accepted it only after the English government consented. In 1841, the English queen sent the sultan a heavy carriage, useless on roadless Zanzibar, but useful to the sultan as a gift to the Nizam of Hyderabad. After some years passed, the English tried again to express their esteem for the sultan. In 1844, they decided to send the sultan a silver-gilt tea service. To the mortification of the consul, when the crate thought to contain the gift was opened in the presence of Said, it held a tombstone meant for the grave of a British sailor buried on Zanzibar. The tea service arrived the next year, on April 1, 1846, April Fool's Day. Fortunately, the sultan needed English support and had a sense of humor.[15]

Overall, the English remained predisposed to a militarized foreign policy after the Napoleonic Wars. In the Persian Gulf area, England found that active diplomacy backed by frequent visits of English warships was an effective cure for the piracy that otherwise plagued merchants and travelers in those waters. During the Napoleonic Wars they had allowed Arab pirates to infest the Persian Gulf rather than risk driving them into alliance with the French. While the pirates might more easily have been kept from the sea by cutting off the timber sold to them by Bombay merchants, the leadership of post–Napoleonic Wars England preferred to maintain open trade and to aggressively police the sea lanes.[16]

Occasionally, England or its minions demonstrated a willingness to move beyond the threat of force. In 1845, English and French naval officers in waters around Madagascar initiated a joint Anglo-French attack on Ranavolana, queen of the Hova people, in her fortress at Tamatave, Madagascar. Long known for her anti-foreign and despotic behavior, Ranavolana had told foreign merchants, including English and Frenchmen, to abjure their nationality and become her subjects or to leave the country, abandoning their goods. The queen's obduracy provoked the officers to an attack which failed. Consequently, her prestige and determination to uproot Christianity, drive out English traders, and protect the local slave trade all increased. Overstretched, unwilling to pay a fine demanded by Queen Ranavolana, ignorant of local conditions, and rebuffed diplomatically, the English government finally allowed merchants on Mauritius to apologize and pay a substantial fine on behalf of their colonial masters, thereby re-opening trade for English subjects. Gold had proven once again more powerful than gunpowder.[17]

There were of course opponents of a militarized foreign policy among England's civilian population. Many of these were manufacturers. Early in the nineteenth century they began to agitate against what they considered "the Norman feudal caste that had quartered itself on British soil."[18] They never quite carried off the conversion of English foreign policy to a more civilian approach, nor did they carry out the reform of the civil and military sectors that was needed to accomplish this. Clever compromise by the rulers forestalled their efforts. Evidence that gold was more effective than gunpowder was twisted around to justify a more militant foreign policy rather than a non-violent policy. In 1836, for example, an influential English writer pointed with alarm to the "astute system adopted by the Russian cabinet. They triumph by intrigue before they take the field; they bribe, cajole and overreach. They corrupt by gold more than they conquer by arms." Other writers resonated with these fears.[19] An inconclusive war with Russia in the Crimea, 1850–1853, was one result of this militarism. A telling indication of how deeply militarized English foreign policy had become by 1850 was the derision with which a select committee of Parliamentarians responded to Sir George Hamilton Seymour's statement, "Certainly I consider that giving dinners is an essential part of diplomacy; I have no hesitation in saying so. I have no idea of a man being a good diplomatist who does not give good dinners." Thirty years of diplomatic experience on the part of a person then England's representative to Portugal carried no weight with the members of Parliament.[20]

In Asia, changes in the English administration of India that began during the Napoleonic Wars grew more pronounced and had profound effects on the prospects for English rule. For nearly half a century between the conclusion of the Seven Years War and the final years of the Napoleonic wars, Indians had accepted English rule. The English were just another group of foreign rulers, though different perhaps in their arrogant emphasis on their kind of order. But like other outside groups who did not bring their womenfolk, they could be entangled and influenced by local women. Indeed, the sexual behavior of English imperialists in India is a classic example of sexuality's dissolving powers and the fear of that power. The Indian mistress, or bibi, grew to have so much influence over the imperialists that some Englishmen felt that "her presence decreased the social distance which seemed so necessary to the authority of the official elite and the prestige of the ruling race." But as communications with England improved, Englishmen increased in numbers and sought out one another's company, most often in clubs, rather than in the company of locals. The exclusiveness of the clubs caused resentment among Indians.[21] Further increasing the isolation of Englishmen was the arrival of Englishwomen to serve as wives of officials, rivals of the bibis, and "the nuclei of inward-looking European social groups in every city and town, as well as in smaller 'stations.' " From 1813 onward, when England allowed missionaries to enter India freely, professional moralists were present to harangue their countrymen into keeping their loins girded.[22]

As the English extended their hold on India, they debated the use of force versus pleasure. Even when successful, pleasure was suspect. Sir John Malcolm received stiff criticism from some Englishmen when he nearly ended a war for central India by buying off the leader of the Maratha Confederation, the Peshwa, Baji Rao, with a generous lifetime annuity. In a letter to the political secretary of Governor-General Lord Hastings, Malcolm defended his action as consistent with past British government practice in India. He wrote that "The effect of this course of proceeding in reconciling all classes to its rule, has been great. The liberality and humanity which [the British government] had displayed on such occasions had, I was satisfied, done more than its arms towards the firm establishment of its power. It was, in fact, a conquest over mind, and among men so riveted in their habits or prejudices as the natives of this country, the effect, though unseen, was great beyond calculation."[23]

With the missionary spirit in the ascendancy and generosity and pleasure in retreat, English control of India became both more direct and much more brittle. The English were increasingly convinced of their own superiority and less in touch with and sympathetic to local sensibilities. They also raised doubts about English fortunes in the minds of their native mercenaries by undertaking an ill-advised war in Afghanistan. Though ultimately victorious, they suffered initial defeats which loosened their hold on the native troops who far outnumbered English and European troops.[24] The Mutiny of 1857, while immediately attributed to religious fanaticism, owed much to English insensitivity and an overestimation of their hold on their Indian hirelings. Eventually a larger number of occupying forces drawn mainly from England, Scotland, and Ireland descended on India and put down the mutiny and associated uprisings.

The increased militarization of English colonial rule advanced the independence of India by many decades in two ways. First, it made the English presence even more harsh and alien to Indians. Second, by throwing more Englishmen into the subcontinent without equally increasing the number of English women, England gave Indian women a much greater opportunity to overwhelm the thin ranks of missionary moralists and Englishwomen. To preserve the distance between ruler and ruled, the English discouraged English soldiers from marrying Eurasian or Indian women. Realizing the inevitability of sexual contact between soldiers and Indian women, however, the British army for sanitary reasons supported organized prostitution. Back in England jealous moralists raged against this and indeed any sexual contact between English soldiery and Indian women. Fear of the bibis' effect on the English soldiery was widespread. By the time Indian nationalism flared up again in the early twentieth century, the bibis had subverted the English hold on India by undermining support for it in England. Thus in contrast to the repressed colleens of modern Ireland, the bibi ultimately undid the empire in South Asia, for she encouraged the colonial to become someone vaguely different and not quite worthy of support in the eyes of stay-at-home English men and women. The latter, of course, wanted no competition.

English civilian leaders sensed that sexuality threatened the distance between ruler and ruled. Indian women were not the only agents who might reduce the imperial divide. When the King of England suggested that a number of Indian orderlies attend his court in England, Lord Curzon worried that Englishwomen posed another threat, because "strange as it may seem English women of the housemaid class, and even higher, do offer themselves to these Indian soldiers, attracted by their uniform, enamoured of their physique, and with a sort of idea that the warrior is also an oriental prince." Another manifestation of the fear that sexuality might bridge the divide between ruler and ruled was the ban on prostitutes from England, though not from other European countries, in Singapore.[25]

England paid a larger price than the eventual loss of India for its use of large-scale violence to hold onto India and for its fear of pleasure. Post-Mutiny reliance on larger commitments of always limited English manpower to hold India sapped the empire. When combined with the military demands of the Second Anglo-Chinese War, it certainly prevented the empire from more effectively supporting the Confederate States of America and stunting the United States before it could emerge as the world's greatest economic and military power. With regard to Europe and Eurasia, generally, as Paul Schroeder notes of this era of Russian, French, and Prussian expansion, "It is hard to find two decades in British history from 1688 to 1945 in which it exerted less influence in Europe or control over the international system than 1855 to 1875. All the major developments of these decades in European politics, and some in world politics, were ones which Britain either failed to control or simply observed without important participation."[26] But Britain remained militarily engaged around the world, consistently winning wars fought for geopolitical purposes, bleeding itself into decline, a victor ultimately despoiled by former victims and jackals alike.[27]

The efforts at establishing racial apartheid by banning all sexual racial mingling affected the whole English empire. "Such apartheid," Derek Hopwood notes, "reinforced in many places by the presence of English women, underlined imperial sexual worries and was at the root of racial antagonisms."[28] Nevertheless, there was resistance that took a long time to die out. In Burma, where Englishwomen were far fewer and the lure of the native women that much greater, there was continuing recognition of the value and danger of the local mistresses to the imperialists. They made excellent language teachers and more. Lord George Hamilton, the secretary of state, recognized that relations with Burmese concubines gave officials "a good insight into and knowledge of local customs and ideas, but there is always the danger that the mistress might take advantage of her position and receive bribes or embark in other illicit practices." While marriage to the concubine might protect the officials from censure, it would lower them in native eyes, thought Hamilton. There was also sentiment that mistresses were preferable to wives, because marriage removed the Burmese woman from all restraint.[29]

In Malaysia, early acceptance of the utility of the concubine finally gave way in 1909 to prohibition as dictated in Secret Circular A of the Secretary of State for the Colonies. Many flouted the prohibition to take non-Malay mistresses from among the Siamese, Chinese, Indians, or Japanese. Taking a Malay as a mistress was banned, especially in Johore State, where the sultan made doing so grounds for expulsion. The sultan's efforts to consort with European women, even to the point of kidnapping, were notorious and a source of scandal and tension. In Sarawak, on the north coast of Borneo, however, keeping one attractive native mistress was encouraged by Charles Brooke, the second British White Rajah, who died in 1917 after a tenure that had begun in the 1860s. Brooke did not expect his young British recruits to be monastic or promiscuous. Furthermore, he "believed that the presence of too many European women in Sarawak would prevent his officers from getting to know the country." In Sarawak, those who learned their Malay from a mistress, locally called "sleeping dictionaries," learned "the language and the dialect very much better and more colloquially" than otherwise possible, an essential factor in understanding "a society bound up with all sorts of complex taboos." The mistresses were very encouraging teachers. Those who learned the language in this way, however, spoke in a manner that betrayed the source of the instruction.[30]

Marriage to native women, though "totally discouraged" during the Victorian era, subsequently became in some places less of a disqualification. Consuls who insisted on marrying local women would find themselves professionally marooned at remote consulates, far from important commercial centers. In China, however, even during the supposedly more enlightened post-Victorian era of 1912–1937, ten British consular officers were compulsorily retired for reasons such as "eccentricity" or marriage to Chinese women.[31]

In the declining Ottoman empire, the linguistic challenges facing English consuls, who normally spoke Arabic if they spoke any language other than English or French, were surmounted with the aid not of wives and mistresses but of miserably paid locals who desired the official protection of a foreign consulate. They subsisted off of private business advantaged by the system of extraterritoriality or, more likely, bribes encouraged by it. Even the consuls who were rather better but still inadequately paid were not above accepting bribes. "In the Ottoman dominions," observed the historian of the English consular service, D.C.M. Platt, "where bribes were the normal path to official business, and where bribery itself had reached such a level of sophistication that it was often difficult either for an outsider to detect it or for the recipient himself to be aware of his own corruption, it was hardly to be wondered at that consuls frequently gave way to temptation. Once they had begun, they found it extraordinarily hard to stop."[32]

Corrupted or not, the consuls played a valuable peacekeeping role for their government, whose main anxiety, Platt tells us, "was that a European war might develop out of national or religious conflict within the Ottoman Empire," much as the Crimean War had begun with such a conflict at Jerusalem. "Consul Holmes argued from Bosnia in 1872 that the most valuable and important function of a political consulate was preventive. With so many different creeds and races, of the most turbulent dispositions, there was a constant danger of collision between governors and governed, and among the governed themselves. This had to be watched, and if possible controlled, since it might at any moment involve half Europe in confusion, and what affected Europe interested England." Peacemaking was an important function of the English consul in Beirut which was much afflicted with strife. And so it was in other commercial centers.[33]

In this age English appeasement continued to be parsimonious, usually concessions of unwanted land in dangerous territory. Commenting on the possibility of withdrawing from Egypt as a concession to the fading Ottoman empire, Lord Salisbury himself noted his "great objection to fixing a date for the evacuation of Egypt, is that relief from our hated presence is the one bribe we have to offer, the price we have to pay for any little advantages we may desire to secure."[34] While Britons hung on in the Levant during the late nineteenth and early twentieth centuries, they began to push into Africa in a way that might be equated to the rush of the Manchus into the disease-ridden jungles and uplands of southwest China. The lust for prestige and the addiction to excitement and the exotic, which was manifested in the decoration of London with memorials, museums, and zoological gardens showcasing the latest round of tropical and subtropical adventures, combined with zeal for gold and diamonds to propel Englishmen and women further and further into the African interior. Eventually individual initiatives brought the motherland into competition with other colonial powers. Ambivalent English leaders were willing to severely strain relations with neighboring France to secure the gains of their compatriots in Africa but calculated that Belgium and Germany had to be appeased with African territory, and so they were.

The decision to oppose France in Africa flew in the face of English fear of international competition, diplomatic isolation, and even a French attack abetted by Irish patriots. In an 1888 Cabinet Memorandum, Lord Salisbury reminded his colleagues that the French could move 30,000 soldiers from bases in France across the English Channel within a matter of hours. "If a Saturday night were selected for the operation," he warned, "and if two or three Irish patriots were employed to cut the telegraphic wires at suitable points after 9 o'clock in the evening, a large portion of the expedition might be one day's march upon its road to London before the military authorities in that city were fully aware of what was taking place. The advance to London would presumably consist of four days' forced marches."[35] Fear of France haunted England's rulers for years and compounded their fear that an expansionist Russia would seize Constantinople, threaten the route to India, through the Suez Canal, and call into question England's fitness to rule India. The very existence of a French fleet at Toulon pinned down the English to defense of their home waters. To save India, England had to be prepared to crush the French fleet.[36]

The adventurer Cecil John Rhodes organized much of the English expansionism in southern Africa. Rhodes could be a ruthless competitor and violent aggressor but normally inclined to employ compromise or bribery to achieve his ends. He hoped to expand England's empire but believed that the far-flung empire was even then biting off more than it could chew and digest to good effect. So Rhodes developed and funded a long-range plan for a secret society, something of a mixture of the Masonic Order and the Society of Jesus, which would work for the expansion of the empire through large-scale British emigration into areas where English was not spoken, draw together the empire, and recover for it the United States. He proposed to recruit this society from the emerging leadership in English-speaking countries, including the United States, by giving scholarships for study at his alma mater, Oxford University, to promising young men with a bent for the rough and tumble of athletics.[37] Opinion makers in the United States subsequently placed great value on the Rhodes Fellowships, and Rhodes Fellows attained high office in the United States and elsewhere. President William Jefferson Clinton was one such Rhodes Fellow, and his political coterie included other Rhodes Fellows, but his stand against British policy in Northern Ireland demonstrated the limits of the fellowship program.

Lacking natural protection against some of the endemic diseases, the Europeans fought and schemed successfully to take over the healthier and more promising mineral land and to recruit as many men to the mines as they could. Greed for land and the underlying minerals encouraged the English to take great risks in fighting the local Africans. But they also manipulated African leaders in the classic imperial fashion of divide and conquer. African military resistance to the advances of Rhodes and other English adventurers was ultimately a failure. The supply of European miners growing too small, the European mine owners recruited as many Africans to work the mines as they could by enforcing the collection of money taxes with fire and rifle. To earn that hard money, African men had to leave their towns and work in the mines. There was some non-militarized local resistance. Ronald Hyam notes of Mr. J. E. Stephenson, as administrator in Northern Rhodesia under the British South Africa Company, that he "was sent to burn down a village in arrears with its taxes and was effectively put off his stroke by the two girls deputed to the task. He resigned, settled in the bush, married three African wives, had several children, and acquired a great reputation as a magician. Although he maintained the white man's dignity, he was never again received in European society."[38] Shades of Ireland beyond the Pale.

Expansion in southern Africa led to war with the Boers. The current of militarism fed by the exciting adventure of the Boer War led the leadership of Britain in a roundabout way to the shambles of World War I and the status of a rapidly declining second-class power. Setbacks experienced in that war underscored the limitations of England's military power and encouraged the militarists to push for a larger role in British foreign policy. The perception of community between Boers and Germans magnified English fears of Germany's increase in military, especially naval, power.

Rather than adjust to the emergence of Germany as a major factor on the European continent, English leaders rebuffed the Germans and allied with the Japanese, and subsequently with France and Russia, both of which had a history of friction with England. The French and Francophiles running the English Foreign Office worked to solidify the new relationship by eliminating any lingering Germanophilia in David Lloyd George, an increasingly powerful cabinet member deemed likely to seek an end to the naval race with Germany. The French president, the French minister of commerce, and the local British chamber of commerce invited Lloyd George to Paris in the spring of 1908. The foreign office advised the English ambassador in Paris, "A pleasant stay in Paris may contribute to complete his conversion and anything you could say or do in that direction would be of great use."[39] The pleasures of Paris in the springtime had a substantial but not a permanent effect on Lloyd George. In 1911, he was in the forefront of decisive English opposition to a German attempt to gain a foothold on the Mediterranean coast at Agadir, Morocco. This preserved France's control of Morocco. But in January 1914, he was again hopeful that England could reach an accommodation with Germany in foreign affairs, a well-publicized view that upset the French and maddened his Francophile colleagues, especially Winston Churchill, the First Lord of the Admiralty. Prime Minister Asquith foretold that there would be a confrontation between Lloyd George and Churchill once the First Lord returned to England from "his Paris fleshpots."[40] Churchill won the confrontation and aborted any hopes of a naval detente with Germany.

As the French used personal pleasure to woo England's leaders, the English leaders in turn tried to use complaisance and pleasure to strengthen their country's diplomatic position. They acquiesced in the rise of American imperialism in Latin America and the Pacific. They cultivated personal friendships with American presidents and influential political figures. The Ulsterman James Bryce, who was England's ambassador to the United States from 1906 to 1913, developed enormous goodwill for England by the flattery of his scholarly attention to American government and society.

He also developed widespread friendships through "indefatigable" personal attendance and correspondence.[41] Bryce's successor, Sir Cecil Spring-Rice, a good friend of Theodore Roosevelt and other Republicans, was less successful in establishing a circle of influential friends in the Woodrow Wilson administration.[42] Certainly the friendships of Bryce were helpful in resolving matters between the two English-speaking countries. The utility of friendship for Spring-Rice is less easy to discern and credit.

Whether accommodating German interests would have averted war with Germany cannot be known, but accommodating two old enemies, France and Russia, did lead to such a war. Cultivation of American friendship, while painful, had less of a downside. Allowing neutral America to sell Germany materials of war did increase English casualties in the war but kept open the door to American assistance, which was crucial to the defeat of Germany. Eventually, the wartime trade with England and France became so profitable that the United States put up grudgingly with English restriction of trade with Germany. The Americans could be bought, while the war's outcome was yet unclear; others could not. The prospects of a 5 million pound sterling loan from England did not impress the Rumanians, who waited for England to show that it could win the war; outright bribery of Bulgarian leaders also failed to win them over in the absence of prospects for an Entente victory.[43]

The Wilsonian strategy of charging into battle when the combatants were near exhaustion helped save Britain from defeat by Germany and gained for America an illusory opportunity to dictate the peace. In fact, the United States did not yet have in place the governmental, social, and economic mechanisms to replace Britain as the world's foremost power. Britain had time but not enough surviving upper-middle-class and upper-class sons pushing outward to make a credible presence abroad after World War I. The desperate energy of years past was gone. There were not enough of the elite left to maintain the old empire, or even to fill posts at home. Labor Party members assumed leading roles. It is also probable that the sexually repressive morals characterizing Britain since the late Victorian period depleted the energies and numbers of the elite and their followers, making the slaughter of World War I all the more devastating to the empire.[44]

The falling tide of British elitism and the sense of entitlement radiated by the British elite and their middle-class emulators contrasted with and in some ways encouraged anti-colonialism abroad. In Ireland, proponents of an Irish republic made a bloody, semi-successful attempt to throw off British rule. In India, in contrast, "despite occasional outbreaks of mob violence and some terrorist crimes in Bengal and in the Punjab and United

Provinces, the principle of non-violence was generally observed." Mahatma Gandhi and his followers successfully advanced the cause of Indian independence with what ultimately proved to be a successful strategy of persistent non-violent resistance to English rule.[45]

As long as Germany was prostrate, England's imperial military strategy focused on Asia. It was based on the hope that England's aggressive ally, Japan, would not challenge English interests. If Japan turned hostile, the English would confront it with their fleet, which would operate out of Singapore and apply long-range economic pressure on Japan. The success of the vague strategy was dependent on the cooperation of the United States. British politicians, however, did not view Japan as a potential enemy and consistently failed to appreciate the contrary, accurate advice of their own military leaders.[46]

During the 1930s, Germany and Italy slowly recovered strength and portrayed themselves as aggrieved nations. Not wanting to be embroiled in a continental imbroglio that would encourage rampant Japanese military ambitions in Asia, England tried hard to keep the peace in Europe. To satisfy Germany, England pushed France to allow Germany to increase its armaments within agreed-upon limits rather than to see Germany rearm unilaterally and in a way that might lead to its predominance on the continent. England and Germany worked out a naval armaments limitation agreement, but France resisted all notion of a rearmed, militarily strong Germany, correctly sensing the vaulting ambitions of Hitlerian Germany to rule the continent. Spurning German offers of an alliance, England nonetheless tried to appease Germany, searching for concessions to Hitler "to induce him, or enable him, to renounce armed force as a means of change. What is odd, in retrospect, about British appeasement," comments R.A.C. Parker, "even when Chamberlain was in full control, is the parsimony of the concessions offered to Hitler. One explanation was that the British thought French obstinacy and folly to be the cause of German desire for greater power, another that Hitler was thought to be a comparatively moderate exponent of German discontents so that the more unquestioned his power the easier appeasement should be."[47]

The English strategy of seeking to limit German military power again challenged Germany's hope to regain predominant power on the European continent. German military strength continued to grow. Alarmed by the rapid evolution of a threat so close to home, English politicians relegated Asian interests to a position secondary to those on the European continent. They sidestepped, however, a crucial decision: align with Japan or build a navy strong enough to defend English interests against Japan.[48] The English developed a brutal military strategy for dealing with Germany. It went beyond starving German civilians, as English leaders had done in World War I. In the next war, England would destroy German cities and civilians en masse with a campaign of aerial bombing on an unprecedented scale. This strategy foreshadowed the human-species-threatening American and Russian military strategies of the nuclear age. To offset any sympathy for Germany that might be instigated by Germany's cultural diplomacy, the English leadership also developed an indirect cultural strategy designed to offset German cultural initiatives abroad.

In November 1934, the English government established the British Council for Relations with Other Countries to "carry on a program of cultural expansion or 'national interpretation' abroad." Its purpose, *The Times* of London reported, was "to promote abroad a wider knowledge of the English language, literature, art, music, science, educational institutions, and other aspects of our national life, and thereby to encourage a better appreciation of Great Britain and to maintain closer relations between this and other countries." At the outbreak of World War II, England established the Ministry of Information to supplement the British Council's indirect propaganda with direct propaganda. In 1940, the council received a charter of incorporation as a mark of its permanency. In its 1940–1941 Annual Report, it explained its role in promoting the constant interchange of knowledge, ideas, and discoveries as "a function of the prudent state." It also defined its task as one of "national interpretation," which it explained was "a happier phrase than cultural propaganda [and] implies the employment by the state, to the national advantage, of the whole cultural resources of the nation." Among its chief methods were provision of scholarships to foreigners seeking education and vocational training in England and encouragement of new or existing Anglophil Societies abroad. It also pursued the dissemination of the council's views and cultural agenda through the medium of a press service and entertainment for foreign newspaper editors, doctors, and educators.[49]

During the mid-1930s, while predatory Germany was still relatively weak, Albion acquiesced in continued German rearmament and was faithless to its Central and Eastern European allies. After Germany had grown strong by devouring its neighbors, England chose to fight Germany rather than to seek peace. It allied with Russia, an ideological foe, sent a large, ill-fated expedition to the continent, and initiated a long-planned aerial war against German civilians.

English strategy for dealing with Germany was as flawed as it was brutal. The willingness to engage Germany in a mutual accommodation alienated continental nations and led to defeats that encouraged Japan to sweep England from Asia. Following an Anglo-Japanese confrontation in Tianjin, China, in the spring and summer of 1939, the English government, under Prime Minister Chamberlain, changed its policy in Asia. England sought to win support from the U.S. government against Japanese designs on its colonial holdings in Asia by resisting most Japanese provocations. This was "the first statement of the theme that came to dominate British foreign policy in the second half of the twentieth century: the subordination of British policy to that of the United States in attempts to exploit American resources for British purposes."[50] Chamberlain's successor as prime minister, Winston Churchill, was an ardent colonialist who renewed the quest for assistance from the United States. He personally cultivated the friendship of President Franklin D. Roosevelt. Friendship, however, was slow to develop and in any case would not have been enough to move the American leader to go precipitously to war on behalf of a colonial power. As a Yankee, Roosevelt drew on a deep anti-colonial heritage. As a Democratic Party leader, he had to be attentive to the anti-colonialism of the many ethnic groups, including the Irish-Americans, associated with the party. Trained in the federal executive branch of government as assistant secretary of the navy during the Wilson administration, he was not willing to do more than try to intimidate the Germans by bellicose naval activities short of war. Against the Japanese, he employed economic measures short of war. The Japanese made ready for war.

Beleaguered by the Germans and threatened by the Japanese, England was desperate for American warships and war material but short of money. So Churchill was reduced to trading away some imperial trappings to save the seat of the empire itself. For fifty American ships and war material, England had to turn over to the United States the naval bases in the Western Hemisphere that had been the linchpin of its colonial power there. But Churchill would not do what Alexius I Comnenus had done in 1081 A.D., when he stripped Constantinople's glorious churches to buy the assistance of a strong third party against two hostile groups of Turks. Churchill held back from liquidating England's African and Asian possessions to buy more American support or to buy off the Germans or Japanese. In early 1941, he may finally have wrung from President Franklin D. Roosevelt a secret promise to enter the war to protect English and Dutch colonies in Asia— the record is neither complete nor clear in this regard. Churchill could not, however, induce Roosevelt to go directly against a large majority of Americans who refused to support a war on behalf of one colonial power against another. Roosevelt was at last willing to engage in war. He was, however, unable to induce England's enemies to provide him with a politically acceptable cause for war. So Franklin Roosevelt persisted in his strategy of providing military aid and hanging back until the European combatants were nearing exhaustion. Finally, the Japanese attack on Pearl Harbor gave Franklin Roosevelt a clear cause to lead his country into war. Though the attack came from Japan, Roosevelt pursued a Europe-first strategy. The ambivalent respect of the German dictator for England, English doggedness, the sweeping military successes of the Soviet Union, and U.S. material assistance and military victories combined to save England.

Post–World War II England had once again lost so many of its upper- and middle-class males that its hold on overseas possessions weakened further. One by one they pulled away. The waste of ever-scarcer resources on the development and maintenance of nuclear weaponry, not to mention the detrimental effects of nuclear development, testing, and operations on public health, exacerbated England's decline. Looking back from the mid-1990s over the previous fifty years, the retiring president of the Royal Society, Michael Atiyah, announced his belief that "history will show that the insistence on a U.K. nuclear capability was fundamentally misguided, a total waste of resources, and a significant factor in our relative economic decline over the past 50 years." He went on to criticize British contributions to the international arms trade "which uses the the scientific skills of this country to export potential death and destruction to the poorer parts of the world, where scarce resources would be better employed on food and health."[51] The English arms trade had earlier evoked similar criticism from the country's financial sector. Asking "Who needs an army?" *The Economist* had editorialized against the sale of arms to poor countries and called on poor nations to abolish their armies. Echoing a U.N. study, it pointed out "that in poor countries the chances of dying from malnutrition or preventable disease are 33 times greater than the chances of dying in a war with the neighbours. Yet, on average, poor countries have about 20 soldiers for every doctor. . . . Of the 82 armed conflicts counted by the [United Nations Development Programme] between 1989 and 1992, only three were betwen states; the others were internal." The venerable publication called on rich nations, development banks, and aid agencies to refuse to help countries spending on arms not immediately needed to repel invasion.[52] Whether England would heed such calls and stop the waste of its resources on the trade in pain and violence remains to be seen.

Reliance on the ability to inflict maximum pain and destruction and on the trade in pain and violence not only hastened England's decline but provided it with no defense against the uses of sex in international relations.

In the 1960s, John Profumo, secretary of war, provided grist for the scan-dalmongers when he established a sexual liaison with a prostitute who was sleeping with a Soviet diplomat. The revelation aborted efforts by Britain to seek a relaxation of tensions between England and its ally the United States on the one hand and the Union of Soviet Socialist Republics on the other.[53] In March 1989, London was agog with printed allegations that a former "Miss India" who worked as a parliamentary researcher also "worked as a call girl and had links with a Cabinet minister and a top Libyan security official." Opposition leaders fretted that this might have established an unintended link with Libya; England had broken off rela-tions with Libya in 1984 after a diplomat killed a London policewoman. *Miami Herald* editors chuckled and headlined the story, "London Broil Follows Press Sex Expose."[54] It may be, however, that the Libyans were using sex to influence British foreign policy; it may also be that this and the Profumo scandals served the purpose of those in England who sought to justify a larger military establishment.

As the twentieth century ended, England held on tenaciously to Northern Ireland, Gibraltar, and a sprinkling of small islands. But it had readily abandoned Hong Kong, its most lucrative colony, in anticipation of pres-sure by the People's Republic of China. Because it had chosen not to de-velop local autonomy and a degree of local democracy that might have soured the Beijing autocrats on Hong Kong, it laid itself open to charges of racism and lack of interest in democracy. As Britain is the least demo-cratic country in Western Europe, there is some reason to believe that it resonated more with Beijing autocrats than with the democratic aspirations of its own colonial subjects. To have fostered a grassroots democracy in Hong Kong would have exposed the lack of democratic mechanism and processes at home and in Northern Ireland. Once again, underlying deter-mination to hold on to Ireland may have served to embarrass English di-plomacy and to demonstrate how threadbare were England's claims to be a champion of democracy.[55]

The fall of the modern Anglo-Norman empire can be traced to a cultur-ally arrogant colonial policy and disastrous military engagements on the continent of Europe. By separating colonial agents from colonial subjects and culture and abandoning its policies of minimizing expenditures of En-glish or British blood, it threw away its only hope of maintaining a vigorous overseas empire. Where once English leaders would have put a wall of guineas between themselves and troubles on the continent, in the twentieth century they chose to waste generations of their young men instead. They had the naval and air defenses and the financial resources to hang back had they so chosen, but they did not. By the testimony of English Foreign Ministry officials, it was the fleshpots of Paris that wedded the key political figures, Lloyd George and Winston Churchill, to belligerence in the French cause, effectively drawing England into the carnage of World War I, the pivotal epoch in the modern Anglo-Norman empire. Ironically, the English as a whole were meanwhile denying themselves the pleasures of sex and did not reproduce themselves fast enough thereafter to hold on to their empire. Thus pleasure indulged by the few and simultaneously denied by the many led to the death of millions and the ruin of an empire. Exacerbating the collapse was the waste of national resources in the development and maintenance of nuclear weaponry during and after World War II and participation in the international arms trade.

NOTES

1. John M. Sherwig, *Guineas and Gunpowder: British Foreign Aid in the Wars with France, 1793–1815* (Cambridge, Mass.: Harvard University Press, 1969), pp. 345–356.

2. Edward Vose Gulick, *Europe's Classical Balance of Power: A Case History of the Theory and Practice of One of the Great Concepts of European Statecraft* (New York: Norton, 1955), pp. 151–155.

3. Ibid., p. 160; Francois de Callieres, *On the Manner of Negotiating with Princes; on the Uses of Diplomacy; the Choice of Ministers and Envoys; and the Personal Qualities Necessary for Success in Missions Abroad*, trans. A. F. White (Notre Dame, Ind.: University of Notre Dame Press, 1963), p. 23 (orig. pub. Paris, 1716).

4. Hilde Spiele, ed., *The Congress of Vienna: An Eyewitness Account*, trans. Richard H. Weber (Philadelphia: Chilton Book Co., 1968), pp. xiv–xvi, 24–25, 74–77.

5. Ibid., pp. xii, 164–172, 258–263.

6. Ibid., pp. 100, 244.

7. de Callieres, *On the Manner of Negotiating with Princes*, p. 24.

8. Spiele, *The Congress of Vienna*, pp. xiv–xvii, xxi–xxiv.

9. Ibid., pp. 81–82, 101, 104–108, 166. Just how infectious the English culture and its distaste for continental manners have been can be seen in Gordon K. Lewis' *Slavery, Imperialism, and Freedom: Essays in English Radical Thought* (New York: Monthly Review Press, 1968). Lewis, a Welshman, pillories the English for being "obdurately insular" yet later condemns Talleyrand as "the aging, cynical roué of the Congress of Vienna" (see pp. 10, 94). Lewis' bias against pleasure is evident in this work (see pp. 231–232).

10. Peter Barber, *Diplomacy: The World of the Honest Spy* (London: The British Library, 1979), pp. 40, 45–46.

11. Andre Maurois, *Chateaubriand: Poet, Statesman, Lover*, trans. Vera Fraser (New York: Greenwood Press, 1969, orig. pub. 1938), pp. 240–241, 246.

12. Charles Webster, *The Congress of Vienna, 1814–1815* (New York: Barnes & Noble, 1969), pp. 187–193.

13. Charles Ronald Middleton, *The Administration of British Foreign Policy 1782–1846* (Durham, N.C.: Duke University Press, 1977), p. 27, n. 94, emphasis in original.

14. M. S. Anderson, *The Rise of Modern Diplomacy, 1450–1919* (London: Longman, 1993), p. 126.

15. Gerald S. Graham, *Great Britain in the Indian Ocean: A Study of Maritime Enterprise, 1810–1850* (Oxford: Clarendon Press, 1967), pp. 169–173.

16. Ibid., pp. 237–262.

17. Ibid., pp. 73–93.

18. G. R. Searle, *Entrepreneurial Politics in Mid-Victorian Britain* (Oxford: Oxford University Press, 1993), pp. 9, 20. Though he does draw attention to the contemporary need to learn French to move effectively in England's ruling circles, Searle discounts the validity of this ethnic characterization of Britain's rulers and ruled more than I would.

19. Anderson, *The Rise of Modern Diplomacy, 1450–1919*, p. 185.

20. Ibid., p. 126.

21. Percival Griffiths, *The British Impact on India* ([Hamden, Conn.: Archon Books, 1965), pp. 202–203. Penderel Moon, *The British Conquest and Dominion of India* (London: Duckworth, 1989), pp. 488–489, makes the same point, though he notes that Muslim seclusion of upper-class women and higher-caste Hindu rules against intermarriage and interdining were insuperable barriers to a true commingling of the Europeans with the Indians. He also notes that prior to the missionaries' advent, the East India Company supported local temples, and its officials, troops, and military bands attended and participated in temple festivals, to the delight of all and sundry. The missionaries eventually effected a legal prohibition against this as well as against Company management of religious endowments. In this and other ways, they forced a wedge between European and Indian societies, thereby weakening the British hold on the subcontinent by frittering away the strength their compatriots accrued by pleasing the Indians.

22. Kenneth Ballhatchet, *Race, Sex, and Class under the Raj: Imperial Attitudes and Policies and Their Critics, 1793–1905* (New York: St. Martin's Press, 1980), p. 144. Indians, however, often found the behavior of European women repulsive. As Shelford Bidwell notes, "Indians of both creeds were deeply shocked by European women who were allowed to go abroad unveiled, to meet other men, to eat in mixed company half-naked and even, it was said with horror, to *dance in public*" (emphasis in original). See Shelford Bidwell, *Swords for Hire: European Mercenaries in Eighteenth-Century India* (London: John Murray, 1971), p. 128.

23. Moon, *The British Conquest and Dominion of India*, p. 408.

24. Ibid., p. 671.

25. Ballhatchet, *Race, Sex, and Class under the Raj*, p. 119; Charles Allen, ed., with Michael Mason, *Tales from the South China Seas: Images of the British in South-East Asia in the Twentieth Century* (London: Futura Publications, 1990), p. 65.

26. Paul Schroeder, "Historical Reality vs. Neo-Realist Theory," *International Security* 19:1 (Summer 1994), pp. 144–145.

27. William Bunge, *Nuclear War Atlas* (Oxford: Basil Blackwell, 1988), p. 80, argues that Britain might still be paramount if it had let go of its empire in 1870 instead of consistently fighting, and winning, wars for over two centuries. "Perhaps it is war itself, not victory or defeat, that saps countries," he suggests.

28. Derek Hopwood, *Sexual Encounters in the Middle East: The British, the French, and the Arabs* (Reading, England: Ithaca Press, 1999), pp. 54–55.

29. Ballhatchet, *Race, Sex, and Class under the Raj*, pp. 150–151.

30. Allen, *Tales from the South China Seas*, pp. 50, 124–125, 83, 100–101, 151–152.

31. D.C.M. Platt, *The Cinderella Service: British Consuls since 1825* (London: Longman, 1971), p. 197.

32. Ibid., pp. 159–163.

33. Ibid., pp. 133–135.

34. C. J. Lowe, *The Reluctant Imperialists: British Foreign Policy 1878–1902* (New York: Macmillan, 1969), p. 96.

35. Ibid., pp. 345–346.

36. Ibid., pp. 355–361.

37. Robert I. Rotberg, with the collaboration of Miles F. Shore, *The Founder: Cecil Rhodes and the Pursuit of Power* (New York: Oxford University Press, 1988), pp. 101–102, 663. See also index entry under "Confession of Faith," p. 792.

38. Ronald Hyam, "Empire and Sexual Opportunity," *The Journal of Imperial and Commonwealth History* 14 (January 1986), p. 62.

39. Michael G. Fry, *Lloyd George and Foreign Policy: Vol. 1, The Education of a Statesman: 1890–1916* (Montreal: McGill–Queen's University Press, 1977), pp. 82–83.

40. Ibid., pp. 174–175.

41. P.A.R. Calvert, "Great Britain and the New World, 1905–1914," in F. H. Hinsley, ed., *British Foreign Policy under Sir Edward Grey* (Cambridge: Cambridge University Press, 1977), p. 383.

42. Zara Steiner, "The Foreign Office under Sir Edward Grey, 1905–1914," in Hinsley, ed., *British Foreign Policy under Sir Edward Grey*, p. 42.

43. Fry, *Lloyd George and Foreign Policy*, p. 268.

44. Ronald Hyam, *Empire and Sexuality: The British Experience* (Manchester, England: Manchester University Press; New York: St. Martin's Press, 1990), p. 10, n. 31, adduces historian A.J.P. Taylor's observation in *English History, 1914–45* (Oxford and New York: Oxford University Press, 1965), p. 166, that the restraint

of the twentieth-century English "in their private lives may well have contributed to their lack of enterprise elsewhere."

45. Moon, *The British Conquest and Dominion of India*, pp. 1043–1044.

46. Paul Haggie, *Britannia at Bay: The Defence of the British Empire against Japan, 1931–1941* (Oxford: Clarendon Press, 1981), pp. 11–12, 15.

47. R.A.C. Parker, *Chamberlain and Appeasement: British Policy and the Coming of the Second World War* (New York: St. Martin's Press, 1993), pp. 23–24.

48. Ibid., p. 73.

49. Ruth Emily McMurry and Muna Lee, *The Cultural Approach: Another Way in International Relations* (Chapel Hill: University of North Carolina Press, 1947; reprint, Port Washington, N.Y.: Kennikat Press, 1972), pp. 138–139, 148–157.

50. Parker, *Chamberlain and Appeasement*, p. 260.

51. Alina Tugend, "Respected British Mathematician Takes on Nuclear-Weapons Industry," *The Chronicle of Higher Education*, April 19, 1996, p. A54.

52. "Who Needs an Army?" *The Economist*, June 4, 1994, pp. 16–18.

53. Peter Dale Scott, *Deep Politics and the Death of JFK* (Berkeley: University of California Press, 1993), pp. 228–232.

54. "London Broil Follows Press Sex Expose," *Miami Herald*, March 19, 1989, p. 3A.

55. Tony Bunyan, *The History and Practice of the Political Police in England* (London: Quartet, 1977), is a useful overview of the response of state agencies to political opposition.

8

Whiskey versus Rum: The Roots of America's Bicultural Foreign Policy

The United States emerged out of the English empire and resembled imperial England in some profound ways, including divisions between English sub-groups. The overarching Anglo-American culture, however, had a common political tradition of systematic control and relied on a mixture of pain and pleasure to achieve foreign policy goals. These goals focused on the development of America's international trade and finance.

After its victory over the brandy-selling French in the French and Indian War, rum-selling England attempted to reorganize and extract greater patronage opportunities from its overseas empire.[1] Such efforts led to colonial resistance in North America. The resistance grew swiftly into a revolutionary war that reflected on a very large scale the English leadership's worse-case war scenario, with dissident English groups enlisting Celtic and continental allies. (The leadership's worst-case scenario would have been a foreign invasion of England with dissident English or Celtic support.) The Cavaliers of the Southern coast and Piedmont allied with the Puritans of New England and the Quakers of the Delaware Valley. They also recruited the Irish and some Scots in America to their cause. Recruiting the French and other continental nations to their side was their next step. It was an English nightmare come true on the far side of the Atlantic.

The Anglo-American leaders set out to enlist allies. Drawing France into the conflict on their side against England was a major diplomatic objective of the Anglo-Americans. The French government was cautious, so the revolutionaries fell back on a mixture of pleasurable and violent means to hold off the English until the French could be persuaded to use their military might against England. Tempting English forces to desert in return for farms and wives proved useful and drew widespread support. With the English thus weakened, a combination of militia and regular troops kept up enough military pressure to deny England victory.

American diplomats were divided over how to draw France into the war. Apart from Benjamin Franklin, there was only grudging acceptance of pleasure as a useful tool. John Adams initially hoped that trade alone would be enough to win the French to the American side. He saw no utility in pleasure as a diplomatic tool. Even if the American ambassador to France were "well skill'd in intrigue, his Pockets well filled with Money and his Person Robust and elegant enough" he might possibly "get introduced to some of the Misses and Courtesans in Keeping of the statesmen in France," but it would be futile.[2] Franklin, of course, proved him wrong, repeatedly. Chagrined, the jealous Adams wrote that Franklin was "so fond of the fair sex that one was not enough for him, but he must have one on each side, and all the ladies both old and young were ready to eat him up."[3] In his seventies, the Philadelphian marshalled the wit, elegance, attentiveness, and detachment needed to attract the French gentlewomen. In that way, during eight and a half years in Paris, Franklin advanced the cause of his new and beleaguered country. As one of his biographers wrote, "Diplomats have always stressed that winning the women to one's side is a good part of the battle. In the age of the salon, with its delicate network of influence, intrigue, and innuendo, their importance was crucial."[4]

The old Philadelphian was America's most effective diplomat in France, and perhaps its greatest ever. As the Quakers had once recruited the bellicose Scotch-Irish against the Indians, he recruited the vengeful French against the English. The Philadelphian also used his old friendship with the British politicians, David Hartley and Dr. Richard Price, to keep open a line of communication with the English in the hope that a fruitful diplomatic exchange might be born of that friendship.

Arms did not win the American Revolution. New England was a hornets' nest of militia that the British could not campaign in. But England ruled the seas and denied New England badly needed access to its old trade network in the English empire. The frontier Irish fought fiercely, but they also were ultimately dependent on the restoration of international trade. The lowland southerners improved their heavily Irish army and, with French help, stayed in the field against the English. The amatory successes of their seductive womenfolk helped to drive the English out of southern coastal cities into the open, where they were vulnerable to military defeat. But military victories alone could not end the war. Meanwhile, because the

English were offering freedom to runaway slaves, the southern gentry were in great danger of losing the very basis of their wealth. To maintain their comfortable way of life and their dominant position, they needed quickly to stop the loss of their slaves to the English and to reestablish connection with their English creditors. The patriots of the City of Brotherly Love had involved the French against the English. But despite French aid and military assistance and even the threat of a Franco-Spanish invasion of England itself or the Isle of Wight in 1779, the English maintained control of the seas and had enough support on land to harbor their fleets in North America. The war was a stalemate.

It was left to the diplomats to unsnare England and salvage the American Revolution. Having failed to conquer the Americans, the English tried pleasure. When Lord Shelburne assumed the leadership of the English government, it was clear to him that making war on the American colonies had failed. Shelburne utilized friendship to open a diplomatic dialogue with the Americans. He dispatched an old Scottish merchant friend of theirs, Richard Oswald, to open informal talks with their diplomats. Adding generosity to friendship, he offered generous terms of peace to the Americans. His terms were generous enough to split the Americans from their allies and end the war in 1783. The terms were so generous that Charles Gravier, comte de Vergennes, the French foreign minister, complained that the English were buying peace, and successor English governments refused to honor the terms.[5] The relapse into parsimony would come back to haunt England when it plunged into war with revolutionary France.

Operating under the Articles of Confederation, the newly independent nation had mixed success in pursuing its foreign policy aims. England violated the terms of peace by not evacuating its forts in the trans-Appalachia region. It joined Spain as an obstacle to westward expansion. Since Spain had wrested East and West Florida from England during the American Revolutionary War, it controlled the mouth of the Mississippi. As the American population west of the Appalachian mountains grew, the ability to import and export through New Orleans grew in importance to the new republic. Without free access to the sea, the westerners might have withdrawn their allegiance to the United States, so Spanish-American relations took on great importance for America.

The Spanish government had not been warm to the rebels. The Spanish rulers feared the example given by the rebels to their own colonial subjects, so they had provided some money but no recognition to the American revolutionaries. Their caution had frustrated John Jay, the unrecognized American diplomatic agent in Madrid from 1780 to 1782. Jay had left

Madrid for Paris and the negotiations with England that would eventually bring the war to an end. Diego de Gardoqui, a rising star in the Spanish government and its representative to America from 1785 to 1789, had studied Jay in Madrid. He had concluded that Jay, who had since become the American Confederation's secretary for foreign affairs, was vain, a captive of his very beautiful, attractive, vain, and avaricious wife, Sarah Livingston, whom he loved blindly. Poised to leave for his post in America, de Gardoqui wrote to Foreign Minister Floridablanca that, like many Americans, the Jays were fortune seekers. Accordingly, some attention to Mrs. Jay and "a few timely gifts will secure the friendship of both. . . . I believe a skilful hand which knows how to take advantage of favorable opportunities, and how to give dinners and above all to entertain with good wine, may profit without appearing to pursue them."[6]

Once in New York, de Gardoqui plied Jay, Mrs. Jay, and influential congressmen with good food, drink, and gifts. It was futile. When Jay asked for a license to import a Spanish stallion, de Gardoqui had King Charles III send Jay a stallion as an outright gift. Jay was careful, however, to get permission from Congress to accept the gift. De Gardoqui became a virtual member of the Jay household and frequently escorted Mrs. Jay to the theater. But Jay's desire to promote the profitable trade with Spain that brought in specie to New York and other seaboard states better explains Jay's willingness to stall American access to the Mississippi than does de Gardoqui's cultivation of the Jays.

Frustrated by the limitations established by the Articles of Confederation, the American political leadership adopted a more centralized form of constitutional government. The new central government had far more control over international relations than its predecessor under the Articles of Confederation. At the helm of the new government, the leaders of the American Revolution soon proved to be a counter-revolutionary lot. Because they had persisted in upholding slavery at home, they lived in fear that anti-slave uprisings abroad would inflame resistance at home. So during the presidency of George Washington, the United States began its first foreign aid program. It was designed to help the French Creole aristocracy in putting down a slave uprising that began in 1791 in Saint Domingue. The program of aid to enemies of human liberty failed. The slaves won.[7] Moreover, free and slave refugees put a distinct and indelible cultural mark on New Orleans and the Gulf Coast.[8]

The new nation grew and in many ways flourished under the Anglo-American leadership style of the Virginia dynasty and their sometime allies in New England and the Middle Atlantic states. Still, there was a great and growing divide between English and Celt regions. Anglo-Americans inclined to control others. On a small and medium scale, they tried to control European-Americans through indentured servitude and African Americans through slavery. On a large scale, they tried to control the frontiers through grand development schemes featuring well-ordered relations with aboriginals whom they systematically plied with modest amounts of New England rum and other gifts. On an even larger scale, they tried to control the nation's economy and foreign relations through a strong central government.

The Irish and other Celts who were most numerous on the frontier thought and operated on a small scale and resisted Anglo-American rule. For the frontiersmen who came from Britain's Celtic fringe, whiskey distilling was a technology they knew. It is a commonplace that the frontiersmen distilled their grain into whiskey to develop a product more cheaply transported than grain. Whiskey had another advantage. As a form of alcohol cheaper than rum and more potent than apple cider, it could be the more readily given in trade to the Indians for their land. Thus the Irish subverted the Anglo-American federal government's frustratingly slow system of purchasing Indian lands and hurt the profits of the Anglo-American land speculators and rum traders.

Anglo-American attempts to crimp whiskey production provoked the Celts to rebel. They launched the Whiskey Rebellion that seriously threatened the existence of the republic and the landholdings of its leaders. The central government, under the administration of George Washington, responded with force by sending an army to the Pittsburgh area where Washington himself had landholdings. The Anglo-American army smothered the resistance and intimidated the restless Celts of Appalachia and beyond. Meanwhile, the Washington administration dispatched a diplomat with gifts of rum to the Iroquois to keep them peaceful in the north.

Other events on the frontier and at sea also tested the new republic. The English leadership stoked the militaristic climate in their former North American colonies by not fulfilling the terms of the September 1783 Treaty of Paris. England refused to evacuate frontier forts in the Old Northwest and encouraged the aborigines to persist in warfare against the Americans. It also impressed American seamen and disrupted American trade with the French West Indies. Not until late 1794, when they were deep into war with France and the American government had successfully gotten through the Whiskey Rebellion crisis, did the English relent. Then they plied American diplomat John Jay with wine, food, flattery, and some trade concessions. Jay recognized the ploy and alerted President Washington. However,

Jay was bargaining from a weak position. He and the ruling Federalist Party made peace and accepted English domination of the seas.

American accommodation with England bothered America's French allies. French Foreign Minister Maurice de Talleyrand de Perigord decided to make the Americans honor the 1778 Franco-American treaty of alliance. He insisted that they carry French goods, even at the cost of war with England. France began seizing hundreds of American ships. Relations with France ruptured. The United States sent a delegation to France to work out the differences between the two countries. Through three intermediaries Talleyrand demanded a large loan for France and a bribe for himself. He showed no gratitude for the hospitality shown during a recent two-year exile in America. His losses as a speculator in Pennsylvania land weighed heavily on his mind. The Americans refused to offer a loan or a bribe. The French government tightened its restrictions even more.[9] An undeclared naval war resulted. The Americans were so successful in the war at sea that Talleyrand soon signaled a willingness to negotiate. President John Adams pursued peace at the cost of his political career.

Thomas Jefferson succeeded Adams as president and put a new stamp on American diplomacy. No president yet has matched his success in foreign affairs. The great author of the Virginia Bill of Rights and the Declaration of Independence, successful diplomat and secretary of state, used gold instead of force wherever possible. Jefferson used both force and gold in dealing with the piratical ruler of Tripoli on the North African coast. He also used sex to smooth negotiations with the Tunisian minister by providing him with a Greek prostitute and charging the State Department budget for "appropriations for foreign intercourse."[10] The third president of the United State engineered the Louisiana Purchase, almost doubling the size of his country without shedding a drop of blood. For this success he owed much to the demolition of Napoleon's forces in Saint Domingue by yellow fever and guerrillas.

President Jefferson's record in international relations was not perfect. Still dealing from national weakness, his administration did not deter the English from wholesale impressment of American seamen, white male slavery. It also failed to deter England and France from molesting neutral American shipping. An embargo on commerce with the belligerents was futile, as embargoes usually are.

England dispatched a Scotsman, David Erskine, to Washington to patch up the differences. Married to an American woman, Erskine wanted peace between the countries so badly that he overstepped his orders. He promised the administration of James Madison, Jefferson's friend and successor as president, more than England was willing to concede. To make that point, England, under George Canning's government, seized hundreds of American ships and replaced Erskine with an irascible naval officer, Francis James "Copenhagen" Jackson, notorious for setting the stage for Nelson's destruction of the Danish fleet in their home port. Anglo-American relations deteriorated swiftly. The deterioration was even more swift because the Americans blamed England for their troubles with frontier Indians. The Americans attacked the Indians in 1811 at Tippecanoe Creek. Afterward, many were ready to fight England in a war that eventually gave America an upper hand in the Gulf borderlands but otherwise proved calamitous for the republic.

After the war, the democratization of American political life continued as the Jeffersonian Republicans displaced the Federalists. The old guard, especially in New England and New Jersey, put more of their energies into commerce and industry. They used the profits to build and endow educational institutions through which they might maintain and extend their influence throughout the country. Abandoning sectarian religious approaches, they stressed character formation in their schools and colleges, that is, the inculcation of "certain standards of behavior and modes of self-control." By providing college professors and schoolteachers to institutions throughout the land and training many students from other regions, these states developed political influence and commercial networks that were effective over vast distances.[11] In generations to come, Anglo-Americans would extend this style of building and maintaining influence to foreign affairs. Their cultural approach would complement military approaches to American foreign affairs. It hearkened back to the Byzantine empire's reliance on the Orthodox Christian Church to expand its sphere of influence and to the Chinese practice of using education to solidify control of frontier areas.

Lust for land prompted the ouster of Indians from Georgia and subsequently drew the United States into conflict with Mexico. The American government sought to bribe exiled Mexican leader Antonio Lopez de Santa Anna into cooperating. He turned, however, and sought to lure away the many foreign German and Irish Catholic soldiers in the American forces sent against Mexico by appealing to their conscience and their self-interest. Reminiscent of the American appeal to the Hessians without, however, the aggressive use of sex, Santa Anna in a number of broadsides offered homes, farms, and happiness in a free land to the American troops, including the mercenaries they employed. Mexican promises and the hardships of war led to the desertion of 9,207 U.S. soldiers, including 5,331 regular troops and 3,876 volunteers, nearly a fourth of the 39,197 American casualties from all causes.[12] But the prospects of pleasure and good fortune as Mexican citizens were not powerful enough to cripple the American invasion. The gringos fought and won so decisively that they almost destroyed the very government they needed to treat with. Fortunately, a persistent American diplomat, Nicholas Trist, defied orders to return home. As Julius Caesar had escaped the morass of warfare in Gaul by heaping money upon the assembled Gallic chieftains, so Trist bought his country's exit and a huge chunk of Mexican territory for $15 million.

The United States would later take over land from Mexico through purchase rather than arms. In 1853, working through Southern railroad promoter James Gadsden, the Pierce administration purchased for $10 million a strip of land South of the Gila River. The acquisition cleared the way for a southern railroad route from New Orleans to California. Secretary of War Jefferson Davis masterminded this purchase from General Antonio Santa Anna's Mexican administration.

Pierce's successor, James Buchanan, was a warm host to officials who came from afar. During the last year of his presidency, he and his countrymen provided a spectacular reception to the first-ever formal embassy the Tokugawa Shogunate sent to a foreign country. After a rousing reception in San Francisco, Japanese Vice Ambassador Muragaki Awaji-no-Kami confided in his diary, "There had been so much that was wonderful and new to us that we began to doubt whether we had not been wandering in fairyland."[13] In Washington, crowds numbering in the thousands greeted the seventy-seven members of the Japanese delegation. Women tossed flowers at the visitors, and the Japanese marveled at the excitement. A few days later, on May 17, there was even more popular excitement when immense throngs of Americans strained to see the Japanese march in full court dress to the White House. "I could not help smiling at the wonder in their eyes, which reached a culminating point when they caught sight of our party wearing costumes that they had never seen before or even dreamt of," wrote the Japanese vice ambassador in his diary. "I might say that the whole procession seemed to the people of Washington to be a scene out of fairyland, as, indeed, their city appeared to us."[14] The ambassadors were impressed that the official gifts they had brought to the president and secretary of state were displayed to the public and sent to a museum where they were held as public property, a fate from which gifts to officials' wives were exempt. The Japanese were struck by the handsomeness of American women, including Buchanan's niece, and the lead role that they assumed at public dinners. They were also struck by the distasteful custom of men and women dancing together. "It was, of course, with no small wonder that we witnessed this extraordinary sight of men and bareshouldered women hopping around the floor, arm in arm, and our wonder at the strange performance became so great that we began to doubt whether we were not on another planet," the vice ambassador confided in his diary. The Japanese left the dance early.[15]

While the Americans never provided the Japanese with food to their taste, they did take up all expenses of the embassy, including transport to and from Japan. They also proudly displayed to the Japanese the technological developments that would rapidly boost the nation's economy and its strength. Unfortunately for the United States, this great show of goodwill had little political impact in Japan. The premier of the Shogunate had been assassinated and the imperial government did not publicize the mission and the warm American welcome.

The virulent dislike of the Southern Cavaliers for the New England Yankees soon manifested itself in a self-destructive civil war. After the defeat of the South and the eradication of slavery, the division between Anglican system builders and militant Celtic anti-establishment types would continue as a major fault line in American history. Lincoln's death, however, put another Irish-American into the White House long enough to make another vast land acquisition. The Polk administration had grabbed at the land of upper Mexico to expand American territory for slavery and speculation. It had also taken Upper California and its ports to advance the global ambitions of Yankee shippers and whalers. Now the Johnson administration maneuvered to take Alaska for speculative purposes and to advance the global economic vision of Yankee shippers and industrialists. The Yankees had great ambitions for the reunited country. The Anglo-American Secretary of State, William Henry Seward, orchestrated the purchase of Alaska as part of a grand design to dominate world commerce.[16] The secretary had spent twenty years representing New Yorkers in the state legislature, governor's office, and U.S. Senate. His political ideology reflected the Anglo-American vision of New England and the Middle Atlantic states. Seward believed that the Pacific Ocean trade would eventually be the greater part of world trade. He wanted Alaska for its natural resources and especially for its harbors that would serve as way stations on the great circle route and were thus the keys to the northern Pacific trade. The Alaskan harbors would be part of a great network of coaling stations that with a canal through the Isthmus of Panama, a massive network of telegraph lines, and a uniform coinage would enable American to surpass all of its commercial competitors.[17]

Seward's timing was wonderful. The Russian government was eager to sell Alaska before it was lost to Great Britain, the United States, or a wave of Mormon settlers. The czarist government was hoping to use the United States as a counterpoise to England and thus be able to expend its resources on the development of lands along the Pacific Coast recently obtained from the government of China. So the czarist government authorized its minister to the United States, Edouard von Stoeckl, to sell the colony.

Since coming to America in 1854, Stoeckl had been popular for his courtly manners and fluent English. His popularity in Washington increased when he married Elizabeth Howard of Massachusetts, whom he described as "American, Protestant, without property."[18] Now he traded on that popularity and also invested part of the prospective proceeds from the sale in those who had the power in Congress to speed the ratification of the treaty in the Senate and appropriation of the purchase money without strings attached in the House of Representatives.[19]

Seward, well known as a congenial host, was not idle either. He had the Department publish a short work on the reasons for purchase. Also, he wined and dined influential senators, drawing down on the huge supply of wine purchased cheaply through American diplomats abroad and foreign representatives in the United States. "Terrapin and Chateaux Margaux will doubtless assist in the elucidation of this already knotty subject," quipped a *New York Herald* correspondent. So they did. And so did the memory of Russian support for the Union during the critical Civil War years, dreams of easier access to Asian and Pacific Rim markets, and of a republic expanding to absorb all of North America.[20] Not until three decades had passed and the next American president identified with the Celtic-American culture, William McKinley, took office would the United States pursue territorial acquisitions on a Polkean or Johnsonian scale.

There was a marked change during the Hayes administration in the hospitality offered to guests at the White House. To keep opponents of alcohol consumption from bolting to the Temperance Party, the president banned alcohol from the White House after the first state dinner. The president's wife, Lucy Webb Hayes, received the praise or blame for her husband's symbolic but practical political action and thereby gained notoriety as "Lemonade Lucy." The couple nonetheless entertained their guests sumptuously, and American diplomacy seems not to have suffered for the absence of Chateaux Margaux or other kinds of alcohol at the White House.[21]

During the first administration of Grover Cleveland, 1885–1889, the utility and limitations of pleasure came to the fore. American Secretary of State Thomas F. Bayard, scion of a French family long intermarried with distinguished Anglo-Americans of Virginia and Delaware, had been a fourth-generation U.S. senator and the nephew of still another U.S. senator. As secretary of state, he rigorously enforced a ban on foreign decorations bestowed without congressional assent in a vain attempt to keep the Ottoman government from unduly influencing the American minister to Istanbul. The minister, upon whose wife the Ottomans had attempted to press a valuable decoration, brought back to Washington a proposal for a treaty that would have eroded American rights in the Ottoman empire. The Germans, however, were more low key and more successful in their attempt to use pleasure to improve German-American relations. At the outset of his first term as secretary of state, Bayard found relations with Germany badly strained. The Germans were upset over America's high tariffs; Americans were upset because the Germans had banned American pork products out of fear of trichinosis. Bayard sent a new minister to Germany, and Bismarck's government took pains to give the American minister, Pendleton, a warm welcome and make him feel at home. Exchanges of symbolic gifts followed between Bismarck and Cleveland.

Unfortunately, Germany abandoned this promising effort to handling relations with the United States. It began to expand its colonial schemes to embrace Samoa where America felt it had important long-range commercial and maritime interests. Secretary of State Bayard sought to preserve at least nominal Samoan independence under tripartite English, German, and American direction. Bayard proposed that no country would enjoy special commercial privileges under such an arrangement. This American position on Samoa was a precursor of the American "Open Door" policy in China formulated by Secretary of State John Hay. German efforts to take control of Samoa worsened German–American relations. Bayard's policy seemed about to fall victim to German naval superiority in the service of Bismarck's aggressive colonial policy and to England's desire to have Germany as an ally on the continent (not the last time that England would indulge German aggression). German plans went awry when a typhoon wrecked the American and German warships in Samoa and forced England, Germany, and America to settle their differences.[22]

In the midst of the long and often frustrating controversy over the Canadian fisheries question, Cupid's darts failed to smooth out the dispute between America and its northern neighbor. England had dispatched Joseph Chamberlain, a fifty-one-year-old widower with many children, to Washington to represent its interests in negotiations about the fisheries. In late November 1887, the British Legation gave a large reception in his honor. There he met and instantly fell in love with Mary Endicott, daughter

of Cleveland's Secretary of War, William C. Endicott. "Once more," wrote
the historian Charles C. Tansill, "the ancient mystery of the way of a maid
with a man was enacted on the diplomatic stage." But, as Tansill admits,
though Chamberlain went on to marry Mary Endicott, he never ceased to
be a stiff representative of his country's, and Canada's, interests.[23]

In 1898, the United States went to war against Spain when two of that
nation's colonies revolted. Filipino and Cuban insurrectionists had brought
the Spaniards very close to defeat when American forces entered the fray.
The situation in the Philippines quickly deteriorated into war between the
Americans, who wanted the Philippines as a way station along the shipping
lanes to China, and the Filipinos, who were intent on securing their independence.

To avert the opening of a catastrophic second war in Cuba against the
48,000 veterans of the Cuban war against Spain, most of whom were still
in arms, the American leadership turned to pleasure. They wined and dined
the leadership of the Cuban insurrection and bought as many as they could
of the weapons of the ordinary soldiers, who were destitute, for a bounty
of seventy-five dollars each. To tighten their control of the island, the Americans broke the local labor movement and, using Cuban tax funds, set out
to reform the island in the American image. Among the various public
works and public health measures, the Americans inaugurated a campaign
to establish a public education system staffed by teachers using American
methods to overcome the prevailing illiteracy. The Ohio public education
system was the template, and Yankee methods were conspicuous. Using
private donations, Harvard University brought nearly 1,400 Cuban teachers to Cambridge, Massachusetts, in the summer of 1900 for instruction in
teaching methods. Two hundred Cuban teachers followed them in the summer of 1901, while others received similar coursework in Cuba.[24]

Things did not go as well in the Philippines. At great expense, the Americans slayed about 20,000 guerillas. Two hundred thousand or more non-
combatants also perished as the Americans put down the Filipino resistance
to American rule. Though the fighting would last into 1905, Theodore
Roosevelt declared victory on July 4, 1902. What made this politically
useful declaration possible was not merely the bloodthirstiness of the U.S.
Army but the work of William Howard Taft, a Yankee judge appointed
by McKinley in 1900 to be president of the American governing board, the
Philippine Commission. Taft had little taste for military matters. Indeed,
when he subsequently became secretary of war in 1903 under Roosevelt he
neglected army matters for a host of civilian projects.[25] But in the Philippines, this predeliction for civilian matters worked to America's advantage.

The rotund Taft, following the orders of Yankee Secretary of War Elihu Root, concentrated on building a civilian-led colony supported by the Philippine elite. Though Taft and his fellow commissioners had reservations about the immediate ability of the Filipinos to govern themselves, they consciously sought to maintain good social relations with them. As one historian noted, "Taft regularly entertained members of the elite at Malacañan Palace, the governor's official residence, and at such functions he made a point of dancing with Filipinas. . . . Taft, interested in gaining indigenous support for his policies, wanted to convince the Filipinos that the Commission would treat them as equals. It was good public relations but not an accurate reflection of the Commission's attitudes toward the indigenous population."[26]

Of course, Taft's approach to the *"illustrados,"* the highly sophisticated Hispanized elite, involved more than dancing with their womenfolk. He and his fellow commissioners struck a bargain with them and kept their part of the bargain by solidifying the illustrados' local authority and even advancing some of them to positions on the Philippine Commission. Having thus divided the Filipinos, beaten their fighters, intimidated the peasants, and co-opted the leaders, the Americans settled down to make over the Philippines. As might be expected of the Anglo-Americans, they emphasized education. Disagreement over approaches and high turnover of personnel severely limited the results of their reforms, but the effort won support for the United States from many Filipinos, especially the poor.[27]

While the warriors spilled blood in this period of expansive imperialism, empires took it upon themselves to overawe their competitors, and their own citizens, with grand expositions of their technological prowess. Much as Byzantium staged shows of its might and wealth to overawe its enemies, so the imperial powers in the late nineteenth and early twentieth centuries hosted expositions. In the United States, the expositions at Chicago, St. Louis, and Buffalo demonstrated the republic's strengths—and its resilience too, for McKinley's assassination at the Buffalo exposition did not slow down American imperial expansion. The Americans were not alone in their use of spectacle for diplomatic ends. France and Germany were active in this way too. Furthermore, the leadership of the emergent German empire actively used culture to soothe American fears of German intentions in the Philippines, Venezuela, Mexico, the Danish West Indies, and the Far East. Thus Kaiser Wilhelm II donated an art cast collection to the Germanic Museum of Harvard, began a University of Berlin Amerika Institute, and sent his brother, Prince Henry, on an American goodwill visit in 1902. While one might argue that these efforts were "superficial conciliation in-

itiatives" far outweighed by German threats to perceived American interests,[28] in fact they did no harm and softened relations between the two
emergent powers. To further soften relations with the United States, Germany enlisted friendship in its cause and dispatched Speck von Sternsdorf,
a personal friend of Theodore Roosevelt's, to be its representative in Washington.

After a horrific war among themselves in which America joined at a late
hour, the European nations incorporated cultural exchanges into their diplomatic strategies. Under Franklin Roosevelt, the United States responded
by proposing to the Latin American republics an official exchange program
for university professors and students. First proposed at the Pan American
Conference for the Maintenance of Peace, held in Buenos Aires in 1936,
the Convention for the Promotion of Inter-American Cultural Relations
attracted ratification from seventeen Latin American republics. This program led to the establishment of the Division of Cultural Relations in the
Department of State in 1938.[29] The division's purpose was to promote
mutual understanding, but its late establishment and early focus on Latin
America meant that it had little chance of teaching potentially hostile governments in Tokyo and Berlin just what a cunning and ferocious enemy
the primary American republic would be.

Using foreign aid and occasional displays of power, the United States
deftly avoided the wars that broke out in Asia and Europe during the
1930s. It remained alert, however, to the needs of its European trading
partners who purchased American goods with profits from their Southeast
Asian colonies. This brought it into potential conflict with the expansive
Japanese empire, which wished to engross all of Asia and its resources. The
Americans built up their armed forces and attempted to deny Japan the
raw materials crucial to its military power. The United States mobilized for
war and was just two or three months from being completely ready for
war when Japan suddenly attacked it and other colonial powers in the
Pacific region.

The Americans parried the Japanese and pursued a Europe-first strategy
against Germany and Italy, both of which had declared war against the
United States in support of Japan. Rather than advance directly on the
European continent, the American government sent its forces through
North Africa and Sicily into Italy, where the casualties from sexual infec-
tion by willing Italian women exceeded casualties from the stubborn enemy
military. The pleasure and companionship traded by Italian women and
girls for food softened the Americans. Italy's subsequent political capitu-
lation brought relatively lenient terms.[30]

When victorious American armies reached Germany, they were violent toward German womenfolk. Needy German women and girls calmed the soldiers and quickly broke down the Western Allied policy of non-fraternization by trading sex for food and other goods. In 1945, an estimated 20 percent of German births were illegitimate, a large percentage fathered by Allied soldiers. The lines between conquerer and conquered blurred.[31] Commenting on the American occupation of Germany, historian Gabriel Kolko acidly remarked, "What the Russians took the Americans bought, until the spoils of war became a common enterprise. In this the Germans sold what little merchandise and honor their men and women had left. Not for the first or last time, Americans discovered that the misery of others could afford them the pleasures and luxuries of a society built upon chocolate and cigarettes if only one were willing to deprive the Germans of what small virtue they retained." He went on to record that as a result of black market operations and favorable currency regulations, "United States troops in the Berlin area shipped out a sum six to seven times their total pay over the same period. The ultimate German overdraft in this form cost the United States Treasury $271 million before the military stopped it."[32] It would be more accurate to observe that in the Berlin area the Germans bought peace from the American soldiers at a price six to seven times higher than the American government paid its soldiers to kill Germans. Since the U.S. Treasury bore the cost of this overdraft, the Germans made a good bargain. To their great misfortune, the Germans were unable to make such a bargain with the wildly vengeful Russians. "Honor," if worth anything at all, ought never be equated solely with stoic resignation to brutality or annihilation. Moreover, the natural, moral imperative for each member of the human species is to keep the species alive, not to manifest "honor." The Germans, who had forgotten that during years of infamously murderous treatment of their neighbors, finally remembered.

Meanwhile, the war in the Pacific went badly for Japan. The Americans made steady progress toward the Japanese homeland, which they were pulverizing in a cruel aerial bombardment campaign that culminated in the dropping of atomic bombs on Nagasaki and Hiroshima. Also, after the end of the war in Europe, the Russians attacked and handily vanquished Japanese forces on the continent. Russian invasion of the home islands was only a matter of time and could lead, as it had in Germany and Austria, to occupation and partition and probably to the overthrow of the old order. So the Japanese leadership surrendered instead to the Americans and, the death of some scapegoats aside, got what they wanted. Japan survived almost intact, and the American capitalists did not turn Japanese society upside down.

Having built their empire on the bones of foreigners and their own young men, Japanese authorities sought to sweeten the surrender and muffle the American invasion by sacrificing Japanese women. They had earlier been forcing women, generally foreigners, to calm the sexually frustrated and harshly disciplined imperial Japanese military forces by prostituting themselves to those troops.[33] Now the government of Japan ordered all police chiefs to set up brothels for the invaders and mobilized 5,000 Japanese women to serve sexually the American troops. The 5,000 women provided sexual services to the oncoming Americans at a designated bar and cafe complex. American military police kept order in the long lines of American military patronizing the Japanese brothels.[34] After a time, however, the Americans proved even more rapacious than anticipated and forced themselves on still other Japanese women. Rape, robbery, and murder became all too common on the part of the occupiers.[35] In contrast to events in Italy and Germany, pleasure exacted proved to be far less efficacious than pleasure transacted.

Franklin Roosevelt had found it possible to work in coalition with the Soviet Union. Under his administration, America had prepared itself to pursue an Anglo-American imperial strategy. In collaboration with the corporately sponsored Council on Foreign Relations, a bastion of Anglo-Americans, the government under Roosevelt had developed extensive plans to shape the post-war period.[36] By developing and sustaining foreign trade networks, the Anglo-Americans hoped to avoid a post-war economic depression. They believed that generous American trade, economic assistance, and cultural exchange policies would keep foreign nations from adopting nationalist or communist economic policies such as those that had characterized the interwar period. As far as relations with the Soviet Union were concerned, Franklin Roosevelt, with a great deal of support from the American people, had been ready to follow a "sophisticated international approach, which relied on negotiation and detente," and "compromise and concession . . . to reach accommodation with the Soviet Union," as one historian later observed.[37] The focal point of this cooperation would be the United Nations organization, one of whose arms would be the United Nations Educational, Scientific, and Cultural Organization (UNESCO). UNESCO would develop global amity and cooperation, teaching the ways of peace and eradicating the ways and roots of war.

Harry Truman, a Celtic-American from the Midwest, succeeded to the presidency upon the sudden death of Roosevelt. He tried hard and eventually succeeded in taking the country in another direction, toward a permanent war economy. Truman rejected conciliatory gestures by the Soviet Union, which refrained from occupying southern Korea and denied itself the opportunity to join the military occupation of Japan in the hope that the United States would in turn accept its occupation of Eastern Europe.[38] But having challenged the Soviet Union in East Asia and in Iran, Truman was unable to quell the anti-militarism of the war-weary American people as a whole. Homesick soldiers were in no mood to confront the Soviet Union. They forced a rapid demobilization that handcuffed Truman.

The Anglo-Americans continued to push hard for their vision of a postwar world tamed by collective security arrangements, trade, and cultural exchanges. J. William Fulbright of Arkansas, a former Rhodes scholar, was one of those who kept promoting the Anglo-American approach to diplomacy, year after year and decade after decade. In 1943, as a Congressman, J. William Fulbright had been the chief sponsor of the House of Representatives endorsement of collective security. In 1944, he helped plan what became UNESCO. In 1946, as a U.S. senator, he successfully promoted a scholarship program to utilize foreign payments for American supplies and equipment to underwrite student and teacher exchanges. Fulbright would go on to champion the North Atlantic Treaty Organization (NATO) and the Nuclear Test Ban Treaty of 1963. He also opposed the anti-Communist purges of Senator Joseph McCarthy and became an outspoken opponent of the Johnson administration's war in Vietnam, and of growing executive power in the presidency.

There were many others in government, usually leftovers from the Roosevelt administration, who also pushed the Anglo-American approach to foreign policy. Independently of the Fulbright Program, the Office of U.S. Military Government in Germany established a cultural exchange program as an executive branch, a conscious instrument of foreign policy that was designed to serve primarily United States' interests. Its "objectives were physical and political reconstruction and reeducation; and, with changing conditions, reorientation; and, finally binational cooperation and partnership," recalled American diplomat Henry J. Kellerman.[39] After the U.S. State Department took over the exchange program in 1949, it expanded the program and focused on leaders of various sectors of German society, such as education, the information media, farming, religion, public health and welfare, labor, and women. Special emphasis was placed on equalizing the legal status of women and improving their economic standing, their representation in academe, and the effectiveness of their organizations. Prominent American women leaders went to Germany to share their expertise with their local counterparts.[40]

Truman temporarily conceded control of foreign policy to the Anglo-Americans. He appointed a highly respected Anglo-American, General

George Catlett Marshall, Roosevelt's highest military adviser, as his new secretary of state. Returning from China to Washington to take up his new duties, Marshall encountered reporters in Hawaii who were eager to learn if he had presidential aspirations. "I am an army officer and presumably will be secretary of state. And I am an Episcopalian," he told them.[41] Marshall, the self-conscious Anglo-American, gave his name to a European recovery program eventually funded by the United States. He initially called for the plan in a June 5, 1947, speech at Harvard University. He portrayed it as a response to a European economic crisis that affected American economic interests and promised that, "Any government that is willing to assist in the recovery will find full cooperation . . . on the part of the United States Government." In contrast, Truman promoted the plan to the nation and to Congress as a response to a Russian threat to American national security.[42] Rather quickly Truman turned what were primarily economic recovery programs and secondarily military assistance programs into military assistance programs.

By early 1950, there was soon trouble along the Asian frontier. The North Koreans invaded South Korea, attempting to reunite what Russia and America had divided after the war against Japan. The pugnacious, confident Truman led his nation into a war against the North Koreans. Pleasure, however, had taken its toll and limited American might. As Michael S. Sherry writes, "The unlucky American ground forces rushed into battle in July—from Japan, where they had suffered the ills of lax training, alcohol, and venereal disease endemic to an occupation force—shared that optimism but met a superior force and humiliating defeat."[43] When the Americans rallied and advanced toward China's border with Korea, the People's Republic of China poured troops across the Yalu River in support of the neighboring communist regime.[44]

American airpower pulverized the peninsula and opposing armies, but the foe would not quit. The war became a murderous stalemate. Once again, as in Mexico, a president could neither win a war in which he had the upper hand nor bring himself to retreat. Feeding the opposition to retreat were the Nationalist Party Chinese, who hoped that the Korean War would lead to an American attack on China itself, now dominated by the Chinese Communist Party, and their own return to power in China. As noted below, the Chinese Nationalists paid and pleasured influential Americans in order to advance their agenda, with some notable results. But even the army of mercenary politicians and publicists whom the Nationalists recruited, collectively known to contemporaries and history as the "China

Lobby," could not turn the anti-war tide. Pleasure in the service of war and pain failed the Nationalists.

Truman's successor, retired army general and former Ivy League university president Dwight D. Eisenhower, brought open hostilities in Korea to a halt. Eisenhower was more open than Truman to diplomacy. He was practiced at it himself and was acutely aware of the value of personal friendship in diplomacy. He instructed Secretary of State John Foster Dulles to have the new American ambassador to India, John Sherman Cooper, " 'do everything possible to win the personal confidence and friendship of' Prime Minister Jawaharlal Nehru because of 'the amount of evidence we have that Nehru seems to be often more swayed by personality than by logical argument.' "[45] The former general also attempted to use the mutual benefits of trade to draw nations away from the Russian orbit to the chagrin of his designate for Secretary of Defense Charles Wilson, who opposed selling "firearms to the Indians."[46] Foreign aid was another tool used by Eisenhower to win over foreign nations. His two administrations, however, used foreign aid sparingly. Eisenhower sought to encourage the growth of international trade to reduce the need for foreign aid.[47] Aid was given not to make friends but to serve the interests of the United States by opening markets, aiding exports, stimulating investment, and providing low-cost raw materials and essential materials.[48]

To build goodwill for the United States in its competition with the Soviet Union, the Eisenhower administration in 1955 "backed a high-level 'cultural presentations' effort abroad in symphony, ballet, theater and jazz." But unwillingness to engage in reciprocal cultural relations and to open the country to Eastern European scientists and scholars more than offset any benefits that cultural activities might have won for the United States. As a result, a 1959 survey of the American image abroad reflected a negative image of the United States and resentment against "cultural imperialism."[49]

The former supreme commander of the Allied Expeditionary Forces in Europe was willing to use bribes in the pursuit of national interest. In the Middle East, an area the United States considered vital, the Eisenhower administration's ambassador, Henry A. Byroade, tried hard to win the friendship of Egypt's President Gamal Abdel Nasser. The Central Intelligence Agency (CIA) tried unsuccessfully to gain the support of Nasser by offering him a bribe of $3 million. Nasser spurned the bribe. He wanted American arms. Eisenhower refused, fearing that would set off an arms race between Israel and Egypt. Nasser went on to nationalize the Suez Canal in July 1956. Britain, France, and Israel attacked Egypt in an attempt to assert a measure of direct control over Egypt. Eisenhower refused support and rallied the United Nations against them.[50]

Eisenhower expended great care and experienced political frustration in trying to build a well integrated mercantile empire. Congress was inclined to build up the military but to hold back on developmental aid to Third World nations that supplied America with raw materials. In 1958, Eisenhower was finally able to convince Congress to spend more for economic assistance than for military aid. The appropriation of $3.3 billion, however, was $600 million less than he asked for, prompting him to complain to Sam Rayburn, the Texan who was Speaker of the House, that "he could not understand what the members of Congress were doing—to vote extra money for war—and to deny money needed for peaceful purposes."[51] In two terms of office, Eisenhower's administration reorganized its foreign aid program four times and appointed eight administrators. Such bureaucratic chaos produced disappointing results. Not surprisingly, civilian aid waned, and military assistance grew.[52] Congress pushed its militarized agenda more effectively than the Eisenhower administration pushed its trade-building agenda.

John F. Kennedy, who succeeded Eisenhower as president, was very active sexually. He went to bed with any number of women, including the mistress of a leading figure in organized crime. One of America's leading political researchers, Peter Dale Scott, suggests that FBI Secretary J. Edgar Hoover began in June 1963 to leak to the press sexual dirt on President Kennedy and his brother Robert after the president proposed in a speech at American University an end to the Cold War with the Soviet Union. Hoover linked the brothers to film star Marilyn Monroe and the president to the prostitution ring for consorting with which the British Foreign Secretary Profumo had gone to his political ruin that same month. Robert Kennedy coerced the press into killing the story. He also deported an East German woman who was sexually involved with both President Kennedy and a member of the Soviet Embassy. Hoover made sure the matter was covered up and spared Kennedy a sex and security scandal of the sort that had just brought down England's John Profumo.[53] In this way, Kennedy's personal licentiousness may have narrowed his foreign policy options.

Kennedy's administration launched a large, well-publicized, government-sponsored secular missionary effort, the Peace Corps. The American government enlisted adventurous American youth in creating goodwill for the United States through voluntary good deeds on behalf of the poor in non-industrialized nations. The work of the volunteers had a heroic cast. The American government also encouraged other nations to develop similar operations. The good works did earn goodwill for the United States, as did Kennedy's efforts to bring an end to open-air nuclear testing. His administration also laid plans for the reinvigoration and broadening of cultural relations and injecting a spirit of mutuality into them.[54] He was assassinated before those plans could be realized. His successors, Lyndon B. Johnson and Richard M. Nixon, were consumed by a colonial war in Vietnam and domestic opposition to it.

For all the energy that went into efforts in the mid-1970s to curb presidential war-making power, sex and other pleasures still played a major role in Washington politics. At the very beginning of the Carter administration in 1977 another scandal erupted in Washington, D.C. It came to be known as Koreagate. The Nixon and Ford administrations had managed to head off investigations of the seduction and bribery of Congressmen by the Korean Central Intelligence Agency (KCIA). The Republic of Korea was heavily dependent on the United States. Roundly criticized for its human rights violations, the Korean government decided to fortify its position in Washington by seducing and bribing as many influentials as possible. Its main operative was a wealthy Korean named Tongsun Park. Working with him was Reverend Sun Myung Moon, a KCIA agent with close ties to the Nixon and Ford administrations. The hub of Park's operation was the George Town Club, where lobbyists treated senators and congressmen to free food. The Koreans paid bribes as well. They also put a female agent, Suzi Thompson (Sook Nai Park), in Speaker of the House Carl Albert's office as his personal assistant. She slept with Democratic Congressman Robert Leggett. The Koreans compromised so many Democrats that the KCIA, Park, and Reverend Sun Myung Moon and his Unification Church escaped penalty for these activities, and the KCIA grew stronger in Washington.[55]

Finding a loyal, uncompromised seducer or seductress was not easy in Washington. The White House Secret Service and the CIA located and provided young women to visiting governors and chiefs of state. The CIA grew wary of its "sex operations" as ex-CIA official John Stockwell explained, "because when people begin sleeping together they get confused about other purposes." Still, the agency seems to have continued the practice despite difficulties in recruiting suitable volunteers.[56] Adult female and male as well as child prostitutes were also available. There were, however, drawbacks to using professional prostitutes. According to one retired Washington, D.C., police detective who investigated the matter, "If you're an intelligence service, foreign intelligence service, or a friendly intelligence service or a corrupt lobbyist or an organized crime entity, and you want to influence political figures in Washington, D.C., the bottom line is you're all dipping into the same pool."[57] Commenting that "One of the most underreported political topics is the extent to which prostitution in Washington has been the key to ongoing corruption and scandal in that city," Peter Dale Scott has observed that "mob-supplied call girls, with their phones bugged by intelligence agents, have driven the major scandals of Washington since at least the beginning of the Cold War. Scholarly memories, possibly because of denial, tend to be short when it comes to sexual politics. Few now remember, for example, that the first congressional investigation of military lobbying by Howard Hughes, in 1947, drew attention to the women that Hughes' press agent, John Meyer, had "procured" for military men, including President Roosevelt's son, Elliott."[58]

Ronald Reagan, Carter's successor as president, struck heavily at that Anglo-American creation, the United Nations, and the whole multilateral approach to international relations. During Reagan's administrations, William Preston, Jr., notes, the United States "cut its assessed payments to the U.N., scorning the World Court's jurisdiction and the rule of international law. It . . . refused to sign the Law of the Sea Convention after its ten-year negotiation by four previous administrations; it tied votes cast in the U.N. General Assembly to bilateral U.S. aid prospects, indulged in the unilateral use of force in Grenada and Nicaragua, and threatened to leave the ILO, FAO, UNCTAD, and the IAEA."[59] The Reagan administration also pulled the United States out of UNESCO. It was also uncomfortable with foreign aid and inefficient in its use. As it cut domestic support programs, it also trimmed back to new lows and redirected foreign aid programs in the conviction that they merely bought the favor of foreign elites or relieved the poor instead of building an entrepreneurial class that could subsist on its own. Furthermore, the U.S. General Accounting Office faulted the Reagan administration for inefficiencies in its use of foreign aid, the largest portion of it directed to its armed client, the State of Israel. The pursuit of immediate political objectives was compromising achievement of economic reforms, a larger objective of U.S. policy.[60]

The collapse of the Soviet Union encouraged Reagan's successor, George H. Bush, to be more flexible in foreign affairs. In dealing with the Soviet Union, his administration supported a Cooperative Threat Reduction Program that paid the Soviets to join the United States in reducing the number of nuclear warheads. Over the next five years, the two countries would destroy more than 2,000 nuclear warheads and remove from service another 2,600. In the same period, program funding helped pay for the destruction of 378 intercontinental missile silos, 212 launchers for submarine-based missiles, 25 bombers, and 1,331 actual missiles.[61]

For all of its flexibility in dealing with the Russians, the George H. Bush administration remained inflexibly set against bribery in private business dealings with government. Alone in the industrialized world, the United States prosecuted its citizens for bribery in pursuit of business abroad. Its competitors allowed foreign bribery and gave their citizens tax credits for foreign bribes. The practice, for example, survived a challenge in the German Bundestag, so the United States requested the Organization for Economic Cooperation and Development (OECD) to recommend that its membership follow the American example.

Under Bush's successor, William J. Clinton, the American government continued to take this issue seriously. In fact, the Clinton administration found a new role for its intelligence agencies in the post–Cold War era when it committed them to gathering information on such practices. In still partly classified reports, the agencies soon listed international business contracts worth $45 billion lost to bribe-wielding foreign competitors. They also reported that of the 200 business deals in the previous eight years that they had studied, U.S. firms had lost about half "at least partly because other nations were more aggressive in providing assistance. The U.S. government was providing to U.S. firms export assistance at less than a fifth the rate provided by Japan, France, and England to their firms.[62] Fighting back diplomatically, the United States was finally able in 1997 to convince the members of the OECD to commit in principle to criminalize bribery by companies of foreign officials. The organization's twenty-nine members account for 90 percent of the world's export goods. The agreement, however, did not cover bribes to foreign political parties.[63]

Spending on foreign aid and diplomacy continued to decline under the William J. Clinton administration. Overall, between 1984 and 1996, diplomatic outlays had dropped 51 percent, and military spending was fifteen times higher. The drop was especially pronounced during the Clinton years. Clinton even acquiesced in cuts by a Republican-led Congress in funding proposed for the Cooperative Threat Reduction Program. That successful Bush administration program as noted above had been reducing the number of nuclear weapons by underwriting the reduction of the Russian nuclear arsenal while reducing America's nuclear armaments.[64] The director of the U.S. Agency for International Development (USAID) told Congress, "It makes no sense at all for the United States to possess the world's finest military machine, but to let the very diplomatic functions that prevent war

and instability wither on the vine." Congress turned a deaf ear and cut the
USAID budget by about $700 million, or 11 percent. Between 1993 and
1996, USAID closed twenty-seven missions and cut 3,200 people from its
staff of 11,500.

As a result of these cutbacks, the United States was spending less per
capita on foreign aid than any of the world's twenty-one most developed
countries, reported Peter Slevin of the *Miami Herald*. Leading the cutback
was Representative Sonny Callahan, chair of the Foreign Operations, Export Financing, and Related Programs Subcommittee of the House Appropriations Committee. The congressman from Mobile, Alabama, told Slevin
that he expected to keep cutting foreign spending in the face of opposition
from the foreign-policy establishment. "I wouldn't expect them to be happy
about it. Unfortunately, it's going to be cut, whether I like it or not, or
whether they like it or not."[65]

The cuts extended beyond foreign aid to the very operation of the State
Department. In the course of its first four years, as *Wall Street Journal*
editorialist Albert R. Hunt complained, the Clinton administration cut
more than 2,000 positions from the State Department, "reduced foreign
assistance by 30%, closed more than 30 consulates, and postponed or ig-
nored much-need[ed] improvements in buildings and communications. The
U.S. Embassy in Beijing, visitors report, is in dreadful shape—the phones
don't work and the infrastructure is crumbling." Hunt then quoted U.S.
Senator Richard Lugar (R. Ind.), "[W]e have emasculated our foreign affairs . . . and we'll pay a price."[66]

Rather than seeking the global domination of better times, the Clinton
administration was intent on creating an economic sphere in the Americas
that would rival the German-led European Union and the emergent
Japanese-led bloc in Asia. The deficit-ridden government shopped among
several cities the idea of co-hosting a meeting of most of the hemisphere's
national leaders. Various cities competed for the honor in order to advance
their interests in foreign trade and investment and in national politics. Miami, "Capital of Latin America and the Caribbean" and premier gateway
to that region, made the winning bid for the first hemisphere summit in
twenty-seven years.

As did the Byzantines and the Venetians centuries before, the polyglot
people of Miami, which also terms itself the "Magic City," put on a won-
drous show of hospitality for the foreign leaders and their entourages. Urban beautification projects were widespread, and lavish parties were the
order of the day. Thirty-four heads of state and lesser dignitaries enjoyed
the performances of musicians and dancers from around the hemisphere.

Then billionaire John Kluge's 200-foot yacht, *Virginian*, ferried the heads of state and their spouses to dinner at the Vanderbilt mansion on Fisher Island. They dined sumptuously to the music of the United States Armies Strolling Strings and enjoyed $100,000 worth of fireworks from their vantage point at the Vanderbilt mansion on Fisher Island.[67]

Lubricated by the vast outpouring of pleasure, the Summit of the Americas in Miami was generally accounted a success. The leaders of thirty-four nations reached agreement in principle on establishment of a free trade zone from Alaska to Argentina. The conferees also reached agreement on a number of other matters as well. Meanwhile, civic leaders used the event to advance their national agenda, lobbying federal officials for federal actions that would subsequently enrich their community.

Nevertheless, the commitment to concerted action reached at the summit and the festive nature of the entertainment there sharply contrasted to the generally individualistic direction taken by the United States in its international relations under Clinton, as well as with his more sober style of official entertainment. Nowhere near the scale of official Chinese banquets, nor as festive as the Miami summit, President Clinton's official banquets at the White House reflected both the philosophical modesty of a republic in the number of courses and the expansiveness of the American empire in the food and drink. His chefs scoured the empire from the Arctic to the tropics for choice food and drink to delight, impress, and woo the leaders of other nations. When the prime minister of Italy and his wife visited on May 6, 1998, for example, they feasted on grilled Alaskan halibut, tropical mango, and, to appeal to sentimental ties, fine American wines made from traditionally Italian grape varieties. The sparkling wine served for a toast by the president toward the end of the meal was, as had been done on previous occasions, especially sweetened.[68]

The bias of the American government under William J. Clinton toward military means fed efforts to cut the Fulbright Scholarship Program. The Fulbright Program was one of Anglo-America's great efforts to win goodwill among foreign academics and students by making it possible for them to study in the United States. The program also funded American academics and students to do research and teach in foreign institutions, thereby allowing them to share their expertise and upon their return home to add an international dimension to their courses. Celebrations of its fiftieth year were clouded by an anticipated loss of 25 percent of its funding.[69]

William J. Clinton's administration ended under something of a cloud. There was widespread suspicion that the People's Republic of China had bribed the Clinton administration to indulge China's individualistic diplomatic activities and ignore its departure from standards of international conduct established by multilateral diplomacy.[70] The administration stood accused of not having been diligent in protecting the nation's nuclear weapons secrets from the Chinese. It was also involved in military operations in southeastern Europe that some regarded as potentially another Vietnam. Moves were afoot in Congress to cut international affairs spending by 28 percent or more.[71] In constant dollars, the State Department's budget was 41 percent below its level of the mid-1980s. The department was 700 officers short of its staffing requirements, even though some forty U.S. embassies and consulates had been closed since 1992. Many of the remaining overseas diplomatic facilities were overcrowded, deteriorating, and shabby. Morale in the department was low. A distinguished retired U.S. ambassador reviewing these circumstances concluded that the nation's diplomatic capacities had been hollowed out.[72]

NOTES

1. Peter C. Mancall, *Deadly Medicine: Indians and Alcohol in Early America* (Ithaca, N.Y.: Cornell University Press, 1995), pp. 14, 41–45, 48–49, 73–75, 126–129, 137–145, 157, 163–164, 165, 171. Settlers also grew apples to make into cider. See also Peter C. Mancall, *Valley of Opportunity: Economic Culture along the Upper Susquehanna, 1700–1800* (Ithaca, N.Y.: Cornell University Press, 1991), pp. 113–114.

2. Richard W. Van Alstyne, *Empire and Independence: The International History of the American Revolution* (New York: John Wiley & Sons, 1965), p. 87.

3. Ibid., pp. 163–164.

4. Claude-Anne Lopez, *Mon Cher Papa: Franklin and the Ladies of Paris* (New Haven, Conn.: Yale University Press, 1967), p. 20.

5. Van Alstyne, *Empire and Independence*, p. 222.

6. Samuel Flagg Bemis, *Pinckney's Treaty: America's Advantage from Europe's Distress, 1783–1800*, rev. ed. (New Haven, Conn.: Yale University Press, 1960), pp. 23–25, 29, 61–62.

7. Timothy M. Matthewson, "George Washington's Policy toward the Haitian Revolution," *Diplomatic History* 3:3 (Summer 1979), pp. 321–336.

8. Alfred N. Hunt, *Haiti's Influence on Antebellum America: Slumbering Volcano in the Caribbean* (Baton Rouge: Louisiana State University Press, 1988), passim.

9. Thomas G. Paterson, J. Garry Clifford, and Kenneth J. Hagan, *American Foreign Relations: A History to 1920*, 4th ed. (Lexington, Mass.: D. C. Heath and Co., 1995), pp. 54–55. George Athan Billias, *Elbridge Gerry: Founding Father and Republican Statesman* (New York: McGraw-Hill, 1976), pp. 268, 411, gives the

lie to the story that Talleyrand sent a beautiful woman, agent "W," with the French agents, "XYZ," to win over the American diplomats.

10. James R. Sofka, "The Jeffersonian Idea of National Security: Commerce, the Atlantic Balance of Power, and the Barbary War, 1786–1805," *Diplomatic History* 21:4 (Fall 1997), pp. 519–544, esp. pp. 542–543, n. 50.

11. Peter Dobkin Hall, *The Organization of American Culture, 1700–1900: Private Institutions, Elites, and the Origins of American Nationality* (New York: New York University Press, 1984), pp. 89–94.

12. George Winston Smith and Charles Judah, eds., *Chronicles of the Gringos: The U.S. Army in the Mexican War, 1846–1848, Accounts of Eyewitnesses and Combatants* (Albuquerque: University of New Mexico Press, 1968), pp. 431–433, 437.

13. C. Shibama, comp., *The First Japanese Embassy to the United States of America: Sent to Washington as the First of the Series of Embassies Specially Sent Abroad by the Tokugawa Shogunate* (Tokyo: The America–Japan Society, 1920), p. 24.

14. Ibid., pp. 4, 35–36, 38–39.

15. Ibid., pp. 42–43, 49–50, 72.

16. Glyndon G. Van Deusen, *William Henry Seward* (New York: Oxford University Press, 1967), p. 3, asserts that Seward was an Anglo-American with a bit of Welsh on his father's side and only a bit of Irish on his mother's. "As governor of New York, [Seward] worked for moderate social reform in education and temperance, as well as rights for Irish-Americans—with one eye on political advantage and the other on humanity. In the Senate he spoke against slavery—not a particularly courageous act for a New Yorker, but done with enough passion to worry his political mentor" [Thurlow Weed]. See also Ronald J. Jensen, *The Alaska Purchase and Russian–American Relations* (Seattle and London: University of Washington Press, 1975), p. 63.

17. Ernest N. Paolino, *The Foundations of the American Empire: William Henry Seward and U.S. Foreign Policy* (Ithaca, N.Y. and London: Cornell University Press, 1973), pp. 1, 108–117. Philip H. Burch, Jr., believes that considerable Russian money was dispensed to induce the Senate to approve the Alaskan Purchase. See Burch, *Elites in American History, Vol. 2: The Civil War to the New Deal* (New York: Holmes and Meier, 1981), p. 56, n. 74.

18. Jensen, *The Alaska Purchase and Russian–American Relations*, pp. 5, 17.

19. Ibid., pp. 122–141.

20. Ibid., 86–87.

21. Ari Hoogenboom, *Rutherford B. Hayes: Warrior and President* (Lawrence: University Press of Kansas, 1995), pp. 464, 538.

22. Charles C. Tansill, *The Foreign Policy of Thomas F. Bayard, 1885–1897* (New York: Fordham University Press, 1940; reprint, New York: Kraus Reprint Co., 1969), pp. xi–xix, 3–119, esp. pp. xi–xiii, xxxii–xxxvi, 28–30, 59–60.

23. Ibid., pp. 283–285.

24. Philip S. Foner, *The Spanish-Cuban-American War and the Birth of American Imperialism, Vol. 2: 1898–1902* (New York: Monthly Review Press, 1972), pp. 430–432, 440–443, 446, 458–465, 484–513.

25. Richard D. Challener, *Admirals, Generals, and American Foreign Policy, 1898–1914* (Princeton, N.J.: Princeton University Press, 1973), pp. 50–51.

26. Glenn Anthony May, *Social Engineering in the Philippines: The Aims, Execution, and Impact of American Colonial Policy, 1900–1913* (Westport, Conn.: Greenwood Press, 1980), p. 12.

27. Ibid., pp. 77, 123.

28. Richard H. Collin, "New Directions in the Foreign Relations Historiography of Theodore Roosevelt and William Howard Taft," *Diplomatic History* 19:3 (Summer 1995), pp. 473–497, specifically pp. 490–491, citing Manfred Jonas, *The United States and Germany: A Diplomatic History* (Ithaca, N.Y.: Cornell University Press, 1984). Citing James R. Reckner, *Teddy Roosevelt's Great White Fleet* (Annapolis: Naval Institute Press, 1988), Collin argues that when Roosevelt sent the Great White Fleet toward Japan, he was making a significant gesture to Tirpitz and Germany as well as to Japan. Some gesture! The fleet was patently unfit for battle on the high seas, as was obvious when the fleet arrived in Japan, where the Japanese feted it rather than fretted over it.

29. Henry J. Kellerman, *Cultural Relations as an Instrument of U.S. Foreign Policy: The Educational Exchange Program between the United States and Germany, 1945–1954*, Department of State Publication 8931: International Information and Cultural Series 114 (Washington, D.C.: U.S. Government Printing Office, 1978), pp. 5–6.

30. John Costello, *Virtue under Fire: How World War II Changed Our Social and Sexual Attitudes* (Boston: Little, Brown and Co., 1985), pp. 224–228.

31. Ibid., pp. 224–228, 249–254.

32. Gabriel Kolko, *The Politics of War: The World and United States Foreign Policy, 1943–1945* (New York: Random House, 1970), p. 515.

33. Kazuko Watanabe, "Militarism, Colonialism, and the Trafficking of Women: Comfort Women: Forced into Sexual Labor for Japanese Soldiers," *Bulletin of Concerned Asian Scholars* 26:4 (October–December 1994), pp. 3–17.

34. Costello, *Virtue under Fire*, pp. 252–254.

35. Saburo Ienaga, *The Pacific War, 1931–1945: A Critical Perspective on Japan's Role in World War II* (New York: Pantheon Books, 1978), pp. 236–237.

36. Laurence H. Shoup and William Minter, *Imperial Brain Trust: The Council on Foreign Relations and United States Foreign Policy* (New York: Monthly Review Press, 1977), pp. 117–195.

37. Athan Theoharis, *Seeds of Repression: Harry S. Truman and the Origins of McCarthyism* (Chicago: Quadrangle Books, 1971), pp. 29–31, 69–70.

38. John W. Dower, *Japan in War and Peace: Selected Essays* (New York: New Press, 1993), pp. 163–164.

39. Kellerman, *Cultural Relations as an Instrument of U.S. Foreign Policy*, pp. v–vii.

40. Ibid., pp. 95–127.

41. Ed Cray, *General of the Army: George C. Marshall, Soldier and Statesman* (New York: W. W. Norton & Co., 1990), p. 586.

42. Theoharis, *Seeds of Repression*, pp. 52–53.

43. Michael S. Sherry, *In the Shadow of War: The United States since the 1930s* (New Haven, Conn.: Yale University Press, 1995), pp. 179–180.

44. Those interested in the murky debate over the origins of the war and the motivation of the Communist side should consult The Cold War International History Project *Bulletin*, issues 6–7 (Winter 1995/1996) (Washington, D.C.: Woodrow Wilson International Center for Scholars), pp. 30–125. See especially Alexandre Y. Mansourov, "Stalin, Mao, Kim, and China's Decision to Enter the Korean War, September 16–October 15, 1950: New Evidence from the Russian Archives," pp. 94–119. Mansourov concludes that Russia and China could well have decided to let North Korea go under United Nations control had not MacArthur's bellicosity "literally pushed the insecure Chinese to the brink, compelling them almost against their will to intervene in Korea, thereby providing Stalin a legitimate reason to reconsider his own decision to evacuate Korea."

45. Fred I. Greenstein, *The Hidden-Hand Presidency: Eisenhower as Leader* (New York: Basic Books, 1982), p. 78.

46. Ibid., pp. 109–110.

47. Chester J. Pach, Jr. and Elmo Richardson, *The Presidency of Dwight D. Eisenhower*, rev. ed. (Lawrence: University Press of Kansas, 1991), p. 82.

48. William Preston, Jr., "The History of U.S.–UNESCO Relations," in William Preston, Jr., Edward S. Herman, and Herbert I. Schiller, *Hope & Folly: The United States and UNESCO, 1945–1985* (Minneapolis: University of Minnesota Press, 1989), p. 94.

49. Ibid., pp. 72–73.

50. Pach and Richardson, *The Presidency of Dwight D. Eisenhower*, pp. 126–131, 132–135.

51. Ibid., p. 179.

52. Preston, "The History of U.S.–UNESCO Relations," p. 92.

53. Peter Dale Scott, *Deep Politics and the Death of JFK* (Berkeley: University of California Press, 1993), pp. 228–232.

54. Preston, "The History of U.S.–UNESCO Relations," pp. 103–106.

55. Susan B. Trento, *The Power House: Robert Keith Gray and the Selling of Access and Influence in Washington* (New York: St. Martin's Press, 1992), pp. 100–112.

56. John Stockwell, *The Praetorian Guard: The U.S. Role in the New World Order* (Boston: South End Press, 1991), pp. 44–46.

57. Trento, *The Power House*, p. 183.

58. Scott, *Deep Politics and the Death of JFK*, pp. 234–235.

59. Preston, "The History of U.S.–UNESCO Relations," p. 152.

60. U.S. General Accounting Office, GAO Report B-225,870, "Foreign Aid: Improving the Impact and Control of Economic Support Funds," Report to the Chairman, Subcommittee on Europe and the Middle East, Committee on Foreign Affairs, House of Representatives, June 1988, pp. 9, 23, 31, 50–51.

61. Center for Defense Information, *The Defense Monitor* 25:4 (1996), p. 6.

62. Robert Keatley, "U.S. Campaign against Bribery Faces Resistance from Foreign Governments," *Wall Street Journal*, February 4, 1994, p. A4; Robert S. Greenberger, "Foreigners Use Bribes to Beat U.S. Rivals in Many Deals, New Report Concludes," *Wall Street Journal*, October 12, 1995, pp. A3, A17.

63. Neil King, Jr., "Bribery Ban Is Approved by OECD," *Wall Street Journal*, November 24, 1997, p. A14.

64. Center for Defense Information, *The Defense Monitor* 25:4 (1996), p. 6.

65. Peter Slevin, "Foreign Aid, Diplomacy Hit Hard by Cuts," *Miami Herald*, May 5, 1996, p. 18A.

66. Albert R. Hunt, "More Foreign Aid, but Less for Israel," *Wall Street Journal*, March 27, 1997, p. A23.

67. Jane Wooldridge, Fernando Gonzalez, and Martin Merzer, "Work's Over—Time to Boogie," *Miami Herald*, December 11, 1994, p. 39A; Mary Beth Sheridan, "The Spirit of Miami," *Miami Herald*, December 12, 1994, p. 1A; Tom Fiedler, "Protecting Clinton Took Planning, Skill and Lots of People," *Miami Herald*, December 12, 1994, p. 17A; Jane Wooldridge, "The Summit Soirees," *Miami Herald*, December 12, 1994, p. 1C.

68. Dorothy J. Gaiter and John Brecher, "Tastings: Secrets of the White House Wine List," *Wall Street Journal*, June 5, 1998, p. W3.

69. Amy Magaro Rubin, "Fulbright Program Fights to Stay Alive in Face of Severe Cuts," *The Chronicle of Higher Education* (March 15, 1996), p. A45.

70. Edward Timperlake and William C. Triplett II, *Year of the Rat: How Bill Clinton Compromised U.S. Security for Cash* (Washington, D.C.: Regnery Publishing Co., 1998), pp. 215–227.

71. Center for Defense Information, *The Defense Monitor* 28:2 (1999), pp. 3–4.

72. William C. Harrop, "The Infrastructure of American Diplomacy," *American Diplomacy* 5:3 (Summer 2000), http://www.unc.edu/depts/diplomat/AD_issues/am-dipl_16/harrop_rand1.html.

9

Sweet and Sour:
China Deals with the Modern West

Little changed in Chinese dealings with outsiders when the Manchus formally began their rule in 1644. The new dynasts went on to repeat the disastrously expensive Han and Tang policy of expanding China's frontiers to the south and west. China's costly expansion to the malarial southwest and west brought it into extensive contact with Muslim tribes who made rebellious subjects and introduced their Chinese conquerors to opium for medicinal and recreational purposes.[1] To the very end of the dynasty, despite foreign encroachments on the coasts and river valleys of eastern China, the heartland of the country, the Qing pushed forward on those frontiers and in the final years were accelerating their advance.

Generally, the Qing used a quintessentially Chinese cultural approach to absorb the non-Chinese in Guangxi, Yunnan, and Guizhou. Until near the end of the dynasty, they took the long view that several centuries of educating aboriginal men in Chinese language and culture and absorbing tribes from the top down would solidify Chinese rule on the south and southwestern frontiers. Consequently, they counted heavily on Chinese advisers and schoolmasters as their advance agents. But increasingly toward the end of the dynasty they were ready to bring in troops and formally annex borderlands should the native rulers upon whom they had bestowed hereditary title, seal, and official robe and feathered hat resist their "light, intangible, and unostentatious influence."[2]

Absorption of the non-Chinese was very uneven. Where the non-Chinese were receptive to Chinese culture, men and women appear to have encouraged their sons to study Chinese language and culture and adopt

Chinese dress. But tribal women resisted absorption. Indeed, through marriage to the Chinese advisers and members of the small frontier military units, the tribal women seduced them from Chinese ways.[3] Consequently, the Qing lost confidence in its border troops and moved in military units too big to be readily absorbed by the locals. This encouraged military aggressiveness, alarmed China's neighbors, drained its treasury, and set the stage for rivalry and skirmishing among large unit commanders, all at a time when the Qing dynasty needed to concentrate financial, military, and political resources elsewhere to survive.

The Qing made other mistakes, not traceable to the seductiveness of non-Chinese women, that compounded their difficulties and hastened their fall. Early in their reign, they adopted a pugnacious attitude toward most Westerners. They drove out all but a few Christian missionaries who had come from Europe, including most of the Jesuits who, as a group, had created enormous goodwill for China in Europe. Then, at the very peak of their power and arrogance, when the Qing had attacked and alienated their southern and western neighbors, they took a high-handed, tightfisted, and highly restrictive position toward England and other European nations that wanted to trade with China.

The Qing made some critically bad assumptions in dealing with the Europeans. They assumed that denying the foreigners Chinese tea, to which they seemed addicted, would enervate them and make them docile. One Qing high official, Commissioner Lin Zexu, expressed the belief that if China cut off foreigners from tea, silk, and other goods, they would be hard pressed to survive.[4] The Qing also assumed that denying Western merchants the company of women at Guangzhou (Canton) would create such sexual frustration that the merchants would willingly limit their stay at the South China entrepot. Little did the Qing comprehend that the Europeans were addicted to wealth and worshiped at the altar of mammon. The European merchants were monks of commerce, quite ready to forego the pleasures of the flesh for profit and equally ready to crusade against those who would deny them trading opportunities.

In denying the Europeans satisfactory access to Chinese markets, the Qing made the same mistake the Ming had made toward the Manchus long before. Even a cursory reading of their own dynastic history, let alone of Chinese history as a whole, should have alerted the Qing to the likelihood that the foreigners would fight to expand their trading opportunities in China. The effect of restricting markets was, once again, to bring about an invasion by aggrieved foreigners.

Qing diplomacy was by no means a complete failure. Indeed, had the

Qing been as wise handling other non-Chinese as they were in handling the Russians, they would have been in a position to modernize their country and make the transition to a constitutional monarchy. Qing handling of the Russians was almost masterful. The Qing were able to trade their highly valued tea for equally valued furs, and they were able to trade land to which they had only the weakest of claims and no real use for more than two centuries of peace.

After a rocky start involving much border warfare, Qing–Russian relations stabilized and were formalized in the Treaty of Nerchinsk (1689). The dynasty was flexible in dealing with the Russians, because it wished to head off a Russo–Mongol alliance that could cause great damage to its position in Central Asia. It was also well served by its diplomats, worldly wise Jesuits from the West who were able to use the Russian craving for Chinese products, especially tea, to masterful effect in the negotiations. Difficulties in subsequent years were resolved in the Treaties of Bura (1727) and Kiakhta (1728), in which the economic and political objectives of both parties were satisfactorily resolved.

Following the Treaty of Nerchinsk, Sino–Russia relations were to become the most durable and peaceful great power relations in world history. Those relations did not turn sour until the late nineteenth and early twentieth centuries, when Russia sought sweeping economic and political rights in Manchuria, rather than in wintry lands useless to the Chinese. Under the communists, Russia returned for some decades to a policy of friendship with China. Chinese–Russian relations remained friendly until Chinese xenophobia and bellicosity and Russian tightfistedness destroyed that amity in the mid-twentieth century.

Meanwhile, the overstretched Qing had given way after 1911 to a bloodthirsty lot of local and regional militarists, rightly known as warlords. The nominal republican government that replaced the Qing dynasty continued attempts to expand to the southwest and expand Chinese influence in Tibet, even while the Japanese government was trying to expand its position in China's Shandong province. Calling upon the British for help against the Japanese, the Chinese government received a pointed reminder from the British foreign minister that China's sudden decision in 1919 to repudiate its own proposal for a China–Tibet boundary and break off boundary negotiations with Tibet made it very difficult for Britain to support China against Japan. While the British minister to China, Sir John Jordan, believed that Japan had pressured China to break off negotiations over Tibet to draw attention away from Japanese aggression in Shandong, the Chinese were quite willing to oblige the Japanese and risk Shandong for Tibet.[5]

Jiang Jieshi (Chiang Kai-shek), an ally of the most ferocious group of Shanghai gangsters, emerged to lead the largest coalition of warlords. His political vehicle was the Nationalist Party (KMT), and one of his main sources of revenue was the opium trade.[6] When the Japanese militarists invaded China in September 1931, Jiang did not put up much of a defense but traded space for time. Intent on liquidating the threat from reform-minded Chinese communists, but not willing to abandon military means for dealing with the Japanese, Jiang weakened the defenses of Shanghai against the attacking Japanese in 1932. In the following year, he turned over the Jehol province in the north to them while he pressed on against the communists led by Mao Zedong.

The Japanese leadership had started a war abroad, because they had so oppressed their own people that they faced a stark choice between revolution and foreign war. Either they changed their system and stepped aside, or they relieved domestic pressure by sending abroad as many able-bodied men as possible in search of sex and booty. They chose the latter course, and the Chinese, whose leaders vacillated between pacification and military resistance, suffered immensely as a result. The Rape of Nanjing in 1937 was only the most horrible and well known of the atrocities. Jiang holed up with some of his forces in remote Sichuan; other forces hid out in equally inaccessible areas.

On the defensive, Jiang angled for American aid and intervention. The Nationalists had for some time been cultivating the American president, Franklin D. Roosevelt, with special gifts of tea, stopping short of anything that could be considered a bribe but playing on the president's old family ties to the Shanghai opium trade. For his part, Roosevelt hoped to use China against Japan and provided some aid to keep China alive as a foe of Japan. The Nationalists wanted much more aid and direct intervention against Japan, so in 1940 Jiang sent his brother-in-law, T. V. Soong, to Washington, D.C., to plead his cause. T. V. Soong was a master diplomat. His friendly, low-key approach to Roosevelt's circle of officials and cronies was effective. Soong opened his home to Washington's insiders, plied them with Chinese food, and entertained them with games of bridge and poker. Soon the American government began to provide the Nationalist government with tens and ultimately hundreds of millions of dollars for the purchase of food and military supplies to use against Japan, an enemy of America. One of those employed by the Nationalists to make those purchases was Frederick Delano, an uncle of the president. Another was David Corcoran, brother of Roosevelt intimate Thomas G. Corcoran. Although much of the money was siphoned off by T. V. Soong and his circle to the quiet embarrassment of the American government, the Nationalists at least kept up the pretense of belligerency against Japan.[7]

While Soong's skills as a diplomat were great, it cannot be overlooked that his search for backers was playing into the Roosevelt administration's search for foreign proxies to engage and wear down Japan's growing military might. Suffice it to say here that the American aid that did get through to China was not effectively used against Japan or against the Nationalists' domestic enemies, the communists. Mortally weakened by corruption and written off by the U.S. government as a bad bargain, the Nationalists prepared Taiwan to be an offshore refuge after the inevitable loss of the mainland. Nationalist troops massacred thousands of anti-Nationalist Taiwanese. Though it seemed clear that the United States would not intervene to prevent a takeover of Taiwan by the communists, the Nationalists did not lose heart. Drawing on their hundreds of million of dollars in stolen wealth, they proceeded to buy their way back to respectability in America. In one of post–Civil War America's most illustrative examples of the political power of foreign money, from 1946 to 1949 the Nationalists poured more than $200 million a year, $654 million in all, into the formation of what was known as the "China Lobby." Much of the money went into the cultivation of American journalists and publishers. Politicians, labor leaders, and business tycoons joined the group, some of them for monetary considerations. Seizing on the outbreak of civil war in Korea in 1950, this informal group of influential opportunists not only waged a successful political fight to protect Jiang's regime on Taiwan but also prevented recognition of the new regime on the Chinese mainland and embittered American domestic politics for two decades.

The financial cost of all this to the Nationalist regime did of course increase mightily from the Chinese dinners of T. V. Soong in 1940 to the hundreds of millions paid to publicists and politicians by the end of the decade but, as in the case of the Chinese dynasties dealing with the northern and western barbarians, the Nationalists were merely recycling foreign, in this case American, funds. Initially, they were far more effective than the Americans at buying what they needed most in an ally.

The Nationalist Chinese had other ways of manipulating American opinion and government besides junkets, gifts, and grants, and not all of them were pleasurable. To achieve their ends, they traded information with American intelligence agencies and traded on friendship with American officials. They helped feed the witch-hunts of the McCarthy era and destroy the careers of the State Department's best China experts. They consistently intimidated Chinese in the United States, a pattern that led to violence and even murder, and they engaged in the smuggling and sale of illegal drugs to finance some of their operations.[8] What might have been the most important and costly blow to American diplomacy in this era occurred in 1968, when Anna Chennault, a leading figure in the China Lobby, sought to frustrate American efforts to negotiate for peace in Vietnam. She convinced an already reluctant President Nguyen Van Thieu of South Vietnam not to participate in the peace talks that President Lyndon B. Johnson had arranged with North Vietnam. Five years, tens of thousands of lives, and immense treasure later, the combatants finally forged a cease-fire. Ironically, Chennault's meddling was meant to ensure the election of Richard M. Nixon to the White House. Once elected, Nixon went on to make a diplomatic opening to Beijing in 1971 that would undercut and vastly complicate the international relations of Taiwan.[9] The Taiwanese had overreached themselves.

The successor government on the mainland, the People's Republic of China, as the Chinese Communist Party termed its political structure, early on engaged in guerrilla war in the southwestern provinces, undertook a full-scale war in Korea, and subsequently conquered its huge, independent neighbor, Tibet. The conquest of Tibet marked the People's Republic of China as one of the most expansive colonial powers in the twentieth century. After a falling out with its ally Russia, it adopted a war footing toward Russia for more than a decade and eventually went to war with its erstwhile ally, Vietnam. There were tremendous costs attached to these military adventures and imperial expansion, not all of which could be justified as a defense of the main Chinese living area. Large expenditures on the military were only bearable by squeezing the population and slowing up economic development by years or even decades.

While extending its empire and building its military might, the Chinese government adopted an active cultural diplomacy toward nations other than the United States. It brought thousands of selected foreigners to observe elements of Chinese life, carefully chosen to reflect well on the new regime. Exquisite hospitality was the order of the day for foreign influentials. The wonderfully hospitable routine was a silken gauze that effectively curtained off the failing of the regime and gave the visitors an exaggerated sense of China's accomplishments and strength. The cost of the hospitality was high and involved thousands of people, but it masked the deaths of ten of millions of Chinese and the fragility of an overextended, dictatorial government.[10]

By the late 1960s, the government of the People's Republic of China found itself hard pressed by Russia. Following a number of military clashes along the long Sino–Soviet border in 1969, Chinese leaders decided to res- urrect the ancient Chinese diplomacy of using barbarian against barbarian. After a good deal of diplomatic signalling, the Chinese government reo- pened diplomatic discussions with the United States and subsequently in- vited the president of the United States, Richard M. Nixon, to Beijing to discuss a strategic alliance against Russia. Nixon, embarrassed at home by his failure to end the American war against Indochina as he had promised, responded to the Chinese invitation with alacrity. Faithful to time-hallowed custom, the Chinese gave him a royal but somewhat cool reception befitting a neighbor who had not yet proven himself a faithful client.

President Nixon and his precursor, Henry Kissinger, both took great pride in reopening relations between China and the United States. The ur- bane Chinese Premier Zhou Enlai dazzled Kissinger, whose infatuation with the premier was nearly as limitless as his ignorance of China. Kissinger would visit China often. At the arrival night banquet during his 1973 trip, Kissinger toasted Zhou Enlai: "None of us who took the trip can ever forget the sense of excitement on entering China for the first time, and we thought it was a mysterious country until the Prime Minister pointed out it was more of our ignorance than China's mystery."[11]

Kissinger's China visits, other than perhaps his long discussions with Zhou, were tightly controlled in eight-minute segments. Impressed by the control of visitors, Kissinger ordered the U.S. State Department to make a study of the Chinese protocol office. The Chinese, for example, had gone out of their way to give President Nixon a favorable impression of the Chinese economy by giving Chinese children at the Great Wall toys and transistor radios to use while Nixon was there in 1972. They later were observed collecting them, and Zhou admitted to reporters that the Chinese were trying to make a good impression on their American guests.[12]

Kissinger recalled that "Every visit to China was like a carefully re- hearsed play in which nothing was accidental and yet everything appeared spontaneous." Chinese ability to recall details of conversations with any of the American party "gave the encounters both an exhilarating and occa- sionally a slightly ominous quality. It engendered a combination of awe and sense of impotence at so much discipline and dedication—not unusual in the encounter of foreigners with Chinese culture." Kissinger character- ized the Chinese style of diplomacy as "insinuating." "The Chinese use friendship as a halter in advance of negotiation," observed Kissinger. "By admitting the interlocutor to at least the appearance of personal intimacy, a subtle restraint is placed on the claims he can put forward." Kissinger also viewed the elaborate hospitality extended to him on his first visit as a test case during which the Chinese studied timing and security precautions and American behavior in the presence of the wonders of Chinese history. The Chinese wanted to use "the majesty of their civilization and the elegance of their manners to leave an impression that nothing was more natural than an increasingly intimate relationship between the world's most avowedly revolutionary Marxist state and the embodiment of capitalism."[13]

By October 1975, relations between the two countries had cooled as a result of detente between the United States and Russia and failure to resolve the Taiwan issue to China's satisfaction. American diplomats and government officials visiting China found that prices in Beijing's Friendship Store, a three-story department store reserved for foreigners with foreign currency to spend, had risen. The bargains in antiques and other Chinese goods had disappeared. Prices had tripled in three years. With Zhou long hospitalized and close to death, there was less to distract Kissinger from the motives behind Chinese diplomatic activity. Kissinger in private conversations was given to saying matter-of-factly and without rancor that the Chinese were simply "cold-blooded bastards."[14]

The foreign correspondents accompanying the American president also enjoyed the well-practiced hospitality of the Chinese. As might be expected, in their writings, and those of the scribblers who followed them, there was a previously unknown warmth toward the Chinese government that could only be traced to a sense of gratitude and a false impression of conditions in China. Warmth heated into an infatuation that alarmed Chinese officials, for any infatuation is doomed to crushing disappointment and resentment, hardly welcome developments in a diplomatic relationship.[15]

Neither Nixon nor Kissinger seemed aware that Nixon's pilgrimage to Beijing struck a deep chord in the ever-present Chinese historical consciousness. While, as we have seen above, a weak China did deal with foreign nations as equal or greater states, the Chinese had forgotten that major consideration. To them, Nixon's visit appeared similar to that of a client's.

The austerity that marked the communist government in its early years long saved it from the collapse that had overtaken the Nationalists. Nonetheless, austerity eventually wore thin. By the regime's fourth decade, the children of the leadership had come to be deeply embroiled in the national economy, especially as brokers and middlemen in foreign trade. They proved to be highly susceptible to bribery. Indeed, the *Wall Street Journal*, which in 1980 had reported that bribes were not needed to do business in China, reported in July 1989 that "Payoffs, kickbacks, graft and bribery, all of which hardly existed a decade ago, have become a daily feature of doing business in China." The avarice of Chinese in the mushrooming bureaucracy was a serious deterrent to doing business in China and was persuading many foreign businessmen to take their business elsewhere. The foreigners purchasing Chinese products were receiving inferior goods, because Chinese producers made a practice of bribing inspectors of the Chinese Commodity Inspection Bureau to certify goods fit for export. In the past, such as during the Ming dynasty, as we saw earlier, foreigners might have gone to war over such shabby treatment. Now they looked to other markets.[16] The Chinese government responded sternly, executing some bribe takers and punishing others who were caught by some of the 360,000 public servants in the four ministries "regularly devoting the majority of their efforts to controlling graft." But the problem persisted.[17]

The downfall of communist austerity came not from the avarice of officials' children but from an anti-ascetic tradition of gourmetship upon which China had traditionally drawn to define itself and win over its enemies. Banqueting was certainly the main redoubt from which Chinese society launched its counterattack against the foreign austerity of communism. In the words of anthropologist E. N. Anderson, Chinese society has typically been free of "deep ethical resistance to enjoying life." Noting that "Chinese use food to mark ethnicity, culture change, calendric and family events, and social transactions" and that food had a "uniquely important place" in Chinese society, Anderson observed that, "In mainland China where puritanism is enforced as much as possible, the most vigorous resistance to asceticism has not come in the areas of corruption, reducing childbirth, or sex, but in banquets. Chinese from all walks of life persist in throwing huge banquets, and the government's principles count for nothing. This use of food as a social lubricant, stimulus, and marker is traceable to the very dawn of Chinese civilization—and beyond."[18]

The banquet is a highly useful, even critical tool in dealing with a Chinese government or organization. Failure to realize this can expose a foreign government to open ridicule. When the Queen of England hosted top Chinese statesmen at a dinner featuring boiled eggs with asparagus and chicken livers, the Chinese press, for example, mocked the menu. Secretary of State George Schultz earned the same derision for his country by inviting top Chinese statesmen to a dinner of seafood, chicken, tomatoes, and peas. A Chinese commentator sniffed that "By Chinese standards, these menus are at the level of a snack shop. In China, any banquet at any restaurant of any star rank would be far superior in sumptuousness to this."[19]

The Chinese government reaches out to foreign dignitaries through the quasi-official Chinese People's Institute of Foreign Affairs, something

Chinese officials describe as a "non-governmental, non-profit, people-to-people" organization. By covering the costs of visits to China by American Congressmen and their wives and staff aides, it has sought to develop goodwill among persons able to influence policy toward China. At least one trip by a multi-member congressional group, however, exposed Chinese officials to strong face-to-face criticism of their poor record on human rights. Nonetheless, American critics of Chinese domestic policy voiced concern that Chinese sponsorship created the appearance of conflict of interest.[20]

The U.S.–China People's Friendship Association has been the Chinese government's main vehicle for reaching less exalted people in the United States. It was thrown into disarray by the Beijing Massacre of 1989 and the subsequent brutality of the Chinese government toward domestic political opponents.

Notwithstanding Chinese apprehension about overly enthusiastic foreign reaction to Chinese matters, the Chinese themselves have habitually overlooked at least one important lesson that might be drawn from their long history of foreign relations. The Chinese leadership has often mistakenly calculated that foreigners prize Chinese "friendship" or the status of "friend of China" so greatly that they can be bent to the Chinese will if threats are made to deny Chinese friendship or the status of friend. Denial is not a useful tool for governments. Historically, denial of silks encouraged nomadic attacks by those seeking silks. Denial of iron ending up corrupting the borderland soldiers, who sold off their own weapons. Denial of tea had no effect on Westerners who drank tea, other than to encourage them to develop tea plantations in India and Ceylon. Denial of a Russian request in 1959 to operate a military radio station, to refuel and repair naval vessels, and to allow shore leave for sailors in China did not check the deterioration of Sino–Russian relations, and eventually there was a complete break.

Invocation of friendship or threats to withdraw the status of "friend of China" is a contemporary Chinese tactic that the Beijing government has used even in dealings with foreign private enterprises. Like other variations of denial, this tactic has had limited utility and has caused friction in dealings with foreigners. In behaving this way, the Chinese communists show themselves no more culturally adept at dealing with twentieth-century foreign traders and businessmen than their nineteenth-century Qing predecessors.[21]

Just as foreigners resented manipulation of "friendship," some also found the tight regulation of officially sponsored visits unsettling, to the point of being counterproductive. Visiting English teacher, Rosemary Mahoney, wrote of one such officially sponsored tour in Hangzhou in the mid-1980s. "With these tours, the Chinese seemed to be saying, 'We have nothing to hide,' but the actual proceedings were so formal, so tightly scripted and constrained, that they inspired the opposite effect, and the visitor was left wondering what, exactly, was being hidden here."[22]

The long-term prospects for mainland China are somewhat grim. The greatest threat to China comes from the central government's political adventurism, not from commonly cited problems such as great population size, ecological damage, or political dictatorship. Historically, Chinese governments have made territorial claims so extravagant that they are fanciful. Pursuit of those claims has contributed to the downfall of dynasty after dynasty. The People's Republic has entertained and on occasion succumbed to the imperial temptation. The south and southwest have always been a special attraction, and thus a problem for governments of China because, other than the Tibetan Plateau and the Himalayas beyond them, there is no massive barrier to Chinese expansion. While in recent years the Chinese government has been able to reach amicable border settlements with some of its southern neighbors, it has clashed with its southern neighbor, Vietnam, on land and sea. Its claims to the South China Sea put it at odds with other nations besides Vietnam. Yet for all of the Chinese insistence on claims in the South China Sea, there are very mixed opinions about potential undersea oil and gas in that area, and any treasures mined from there may not be worth the diplomatic and military costs of pressing the claims.[23] Even the current southern borderlands are of dubious value and a drain on the country. Tibet, though barren and desperately poor, has been the object of a long and bloody occupation. As late as the 1980s, the southwestern provinces of Guizhou, Guangxi, and Yunnan were extremely poor and had extensive areas where the average annual income was less than U.S.$40, one-third the Chinese average. Despite stern police measures, Yunnan has become an important pathway for Burmese heroin on its way to Europe and North America. The stern measures have also failed to curb local heroin addiction, with its attendant threat of an epidemic of AIDS.[24] The lawful and extensively negotiated reclamation of rich and vibrant Hong Kong in 1997 appears in stark contrast to these speculative expansions and claims. But fear that the local people would use sex and other pleasures against Beijing gnawed at the central government. The Beijing government planned to indoctrinate the troops to be stationed there with lessons on "the dangers of fast women and fast money" and to warn them against accepting gifts or contacting foreigners.[25] Apparently undaunted by this host of problems to the south, China may have also hinted about extending itself northward. Reportedly, in March 1992, the Chinese Ministry of State Security circulated a claim to all of the independent state of Mongolia and the Mongol-inhabited area of Russia.[26]

Taiwan, a compact island nation with only a few island outposts, calling itself the Republic of China, prospered immensely, even without formal ties to the United Nations and the United States. It spent money for influence. Beginning in 1977, for example, it retained as an agent at $5,000 per month the public relations firm of Michael Deaver and Peter Hannaford. During the 1970s, Deaver and Hannaford were the managers of ex-California governor and Republican Party presidential hopeful Ronald Reagan. Their firm marketed his newspaper columns and radio broadcasts. A staunch anti-communist since the 1940s, Reagan encouraged the Deaver–Hannaford relationship with Taiwan. Reagan visited Taiwan in 1978 and met with Taiwan President Jiang Jingguo. Thereafter, he broadcast attacks on the establishment by the Carter administration of formal diplomatic relations with the regime in Beijing. Reagan won the presidency in 1980. Deaver, who had seen to paying the bills for Reagan for nearly a decade—Reagan had not carried money since leaving the governorship—became one of his three top staff members. He occupied the office next to Reagan and controlled his appointments. The Reagan administration did all that it could for Taiwan. While unable to establish formal relations with Taiwan, the Reagan administration did sell it advanced fighter airplanes, parts, and co-production technology. This greatly displeased the regime in Beijing and encouraged detente between Russia and China.[27]

For Taiwan, trade with America was utterly essential and extremely lucrative, accounting for one-third of its exports and $40 billion overall in 1988. By 1994, its 21 million people were buying $17 billion worth of American goods, about twice the amount purchased by the population of mainland China, which was fifty-five times larger. Repeating earlier successful barbarian management strategies, the Chinese of Taiwan plowed the profits of the American trade into pleasuring American leaders and influentials. They built on the successes of the China Lobby of the previous generation in swaying the Congress of the United States, and indeed a wide range of potentially influential citizens, including hundreds of college professors. Their hospitality on four occasions to Governor Clinton of Arkansas seemed especially provident when he subsequently became president of the United States.[28] Drawing on some of the world's very largest currency reserves, $93 billion in 1994, half again as much as those of the United States, the Taiwanese were in a position to deliver on their promises to

American politicians that they would purchase a lot of goods and services or make large bank deposits in the politicians' home state or locale.

To make that economic message loud and clear, Taiwan put 250 persons to work in its unofficial Washington embassy, retained dozens of well-paid Washington power brokers, supported or had Taiwan companies support Washington think tanks, such as the American Enterprise Institute and the Heritage Foundation, and provided first-class, all-expense-paid trips to Taiwan for Congresspersons, local officials, and other influentials such as journalists. In 1995, it had twenty-one lobbying firms on retainer.[29]

Taiwan's pursuit of favorable treatment from the American Congress was broad based but well focused. A Taiwan business group, for example, the Chinese National Association of Industry and Commerce, paid the expenses of seven House members and two senators who spent up to a week in Taiwan in 1988 for meetings. Six of the nine lawmakers were on committees dealing with trade and foreign policy.[30] Hospitality on the princely trips to Taiwan has also been extended to the congressional staff. One staff member who received such posh treatment told a reporter, "For people working on Capit[o]l Hill, not making a lot of money, this is luxury that is noticed and appreciated. It helped me develop a view. I really didn't know much about Taiwan before I made the trip."[31]

Beyond Congress, the Taiwanese successfully courted American colleges and universities and by the end of 1989 had established 138 cooperative programs with them. Thirty-two states and 107 American cities had established links with Taiwan, and eighteen states had trade offices in Taibei. By mid-1995, twenty-four states had passed resolutions asking "that Taiwan be treated like any other nation." Robert S. Greenberger of the *Wall Street Journal* wrote in 1995 that, "Unlike most foreign lobbying efforts that focus exclusively on Washington, Taiwan has created a far-reaching network of friendly officials by doing favors wherever possible while exploiting opportunities like the Galveston Mardi Gras." Taken along with its handling of Congress, its own democratization, and the improvement of its human rights record, these efforts of the Taiwan government effectively undercut criticisms of refugee Taiwanese that their government was oppressive.[32] These positive actions may prove to be crucial in the accomplishment of Taiwan's diplomatic and national goals, which may extend to universally recognized independence from the mainland.

All in all, openness, fair dealing, generosity, and friendliness with foreign nations and individuals have amply rewarded China for more than two and a half millennia, while belligerence, tightfistedness, sharp dealing, and anti-foreignism have invariably led to disaster and decline. Furthermore, not only has militarism been ineffectual in dealing with outsiders, it has given rise to treacherous Chinese militarists who have been as much of a threat or more to Chinese governments and society than belligerent foreigners have been.

NOTES

1. S.A.M. Adshead, *China in World History* (New York: St. Martin's Press, 1988), pp. 291–293.

2. Archibald Rose, HBM Consul, Tengyueh, Yunnan, No. 15, to Sir Edward Grey, September 1, 1910, British Foreign Office Memorandum, Public Records Office, Kew Gardens, England, hereafter cited as FO, No. 371/865/9058/39165. See also the attached FO memo of November 1, 1910, for an expression of official apprehension about the spread of Chinese influence beyond the limits of Britain's North Eastern frontier in South Asia.

3. E. C. Wilton, H. M. Consul, Chinan, to Mr. W. G. Max Muller, H.M.C. Gen., Peking, June 30, 1910, FO 371/872/32267. Captain Hamilton Bower drew attention to the seductive power of Tibetan women over Chinese men in the late nineteenth century. See Captain Hamilton Bower, *A Journey across Tibet* (New York: Macmillan, 1894), p. 284, cited in Lee Feigon, *Demystifying Tibet: Unlocking the Secrets of the Land of the Snows* (Chicago: Ivan R. Dee, 1996), pp. 89–90. Tsepon W. D. Shakabpa found evidence of the same phenomenon in the mid-nineteenth century. See Tsepon W. D. Shakabpa, *Tibet: A Political History* (New Haven, Conn.: Yale University Press, 1967), p. 179, quoted in Feigon, *Demystifying Tibet*, pp. 99–100. The all-too-common blind spot of social scientists toward pleasuring manifests itself in the work of anthropologist Dru C. Gladney. This lamentable inability to see erotic pleasuring as a strategy for dealing with others leads Gladney to the false conclusion that the eroticism of the minorities is a mental construct of the core Han cultural group. See Dru C. Gladney, "Representing Nationality in China: Refiguring Majority/Minority Identities," *The Journal of Asian Studies* 53:1 (February 1994), pp. 92–123.

4. Lin Zexu to Queen Victoria, 1839, trans. in S. Y. Teng and J. K. Fairbank, *China's Response to the West: A Documentary Survey, 1839–1923* (New York: Atheneum, 1963), pp. 24–26, cited in Rhoads Murphey, *The Outsiders: The Western Experience in India and China* (Ann Arbor: University of Michigan Press, 1977), p. 131.

5. Lord Curzon, Minutes of Conversation with Chinese Minister in which Protest Was Entered against Conduct of Chinese Government, No. 183 to Sir John Jordan, Peking, September 1, 1919, FO 371/3689/123926; Sir John Jordan to Foreign Office, No. 474, August 28, 1919, FO 371/3689/121855; Sir John Jordan to Foreign Office, No. 488, September 6, 1919, FO 371/3689/126511.

6. Jonathan Marshall, "Opium and the Politics of Gangsterism in Nationalist

China, 1927–1945," *Bulletin of Concerned Asian Scholars* 8:3 (July–September 1976), pp. 19–48.

7. Sterling Seagrave, *The Soong Dynasty* (New York: Harper & Row, 1985), pp. 359–375.

8. David E. Kaplan, *Fires of the Dragon: Politics, Murder, and the Kuomintang* (New York: Atheneum, 1992), pp. 222, 243–245. I would not, however, agree that Nationalist China is "the one foreign power with the longest, most striking history of intervention in American politics." That distinction I would reserve for England.

9. Seagrave, *The Soong Dynasty*, pp. 429–450; Susan B. Trento, *The Power House: Robert Keith Gray and the Selling of Access and Influence in Washington* (New York: St. Martin's Press, 1992), pp. 98–100; Stephen E. Ambrose, *Nixon, Vol. 2: The Triumph of a Politician, 1962–1972* (New York: Simon & Schuster, 1989), pp. 206–216.

10. Steven W. Mosher, *China Misperceived: American Illusions and Chinese Reality* (New York: Basic Books, 1990), pp. 94–118. Mosher draws on Richard L. Walker, "The Developing Role of Cultural Diplomacy in Asia," in George L. Anderson, ed., *Issues and Conflicts* (Lawrence: University of Kansas Press, 1959), p. 45.

11. Richard Valeriani, *Travels with Henry* (Boston: Houghton Mifflin, 1979), pp. 94–95, 103.

12. Ibid., pp. 109–110, 121.

13. Henry Kissinger, *White House Years* (Boston: Little, Brown and Co., 1979), pp. 1055–1056, 1066.

14. Valeriani, *Travels with Henry*, pp. 127, 131.

15. Mosher, *China Misperceived*, p. 160.

16. Frank Ching, "Travelling to Peking for Business? Leave Those Gifts at Home," *Wall Street Journal*, September 26, 1980, p. 34, cited in Randall E. Stross, *Bulls in the China Shop and Other Sino-American Business Encounters* (New York: Pantheon, 1991), p. 58; Julia Leung, "Greased Palms Lubricate Wheels in China: Foreign Businessmen Find Everyone's Looking to Be Paid Off," *Wall Street Journal*, July 20, 1989, p. A10; Jean-Louis Rocca, "Corruption and Its Shadow: An Anthropological View of Corruption in China," *China Quarterly* 130 (June 1992), pp. 402–416. Rocca concludes that rather than being creative, corruption in China is "predatory." He notes that it is common in foreign trade (ibid., p. 410).

17. Arne J. de Keijzer, with the collaboration of Allan H. Lu, *China: Business Strategies for the '90s* (Berkeley, Calif.: Pacific View Press, 1992), p. 185. See pp. 183–188 for a detailed study of the issue.

18. E. N. Anderson, *The Food of China* (New Haven, Conn. and London: Yale University Press, 1988), pp. 244–246.

19. Jianying Zha, *China Pop: How Soap Operas, Tabloids, and Bestsellers Are Transforming a Culture* (New York: New Press, 1995), pp. 121–122.

20. Michael Phillips, "Chinese Government Paid for Shaw's Trip," *Miami Herald*, November 29, 1990, p. 16A.

21. See Stross, *Bulls in the China Shop and Other Sino-American Business Encounters*, pp. 52–57 on ritual friendship, and pp. 163–165 on the policy of keeping Chinese and foreigners sexually separated; see also Ogura Kazuo, "How the 'Inscrutables' Negotiate with the 'Inscrutables': Chinese Negotiating Tactics vis-à-vis the Japanese," *China Quarterly* 79 (September 1979), pp. 529–552.

22. Rosemary Mahoney, *The Early Arrival of Dreams: A Year in China* (New York: Fawcett Columbine, 1990, paperback ed., 1992), p. 158.

23. Stross, *Bulls in the China Shop and Other Sino-American Business Encounters*, pp. 63–66. A review of the pertinent British Foreign Office records on the origins of the Sino–Vietnamese dispute over the Paracel Islands reveals substantial weakness in the claims of Vietnam. See FO 676/85 for various memoranda on the history of the matter written from 1931 to 1936, but mainly from 1931 to 1933; FO 676/98, 120, 233, and 337 carry the matter down to 1937.

24. Jonathan Unger and Jean Xiong, "Life in the Chinese Hinterlands under the Rural Economic Reforms," *Bulletin of Concerned Asian Scholars* 22:2 (April–June 1990), pp. 4–17; James McGregor, "The Opium War: Burma Road Heroin Breeds Addicts, AIDS along China's Border," *Wall Street Journal*, September 29, 1992, p. A1.

25. Emma Batha, "PLA Garrison Warned Against Fast Women, Fast Money," *South China Morning Post*, July 18, 1996, p. 4, quoted in Foreign Broadcast Information Service, *China Report*, July 19, 1996, p. 80.

26. Lillian Craig Harris, "Xinjiang, Central Asia and the Implications for China's Policy in the Islamic World," *China Quarterly* 33 (March 1993), p. 114.

27. Ronnie Dugger, *On Reagan: The Man and His Presidency* (New York: McGraw-Hill, 1983), pp. 35, 371–373, 526–528.

28. Marcus W. Brauchli, "Asians Strive to Get in the Picture with Bill: Clinton Photos, Inaugural Tickets Form Symbols of Power," *Wall Street Journal*, December 27, 1996, p. A4.

29. James A. McGregor, "Taiwan Cultivates America's Support with Lobbying Force the Size of Israel's," *Wall Street Journal*, January 7, 1989, p. A26; Robert S. Greenberger, "Let Me In: Taiwan, Trying to Win Status in Washington, Targets Grass Roots," *Wall Street Journal*, May 6, 1995, p. A1.

30. Charles Green, "Fees OK for Lawmakers to Pocket Could Land Others in Jail," *Miami Herald*, September 4, 1989, p. 13A.

31. Greenberger, "Let Me In," p. A12.

32. McGregor, "Taiwan Cultivates America's Support with Lobbying Force the Size of Israel's," p. A26.

Bibliography

UNPUBLISHED MATERIALS

Foreign Office Memoranda, Public Records Office, Kew Gardens, England.

PUBLISHED MATERIALS

Adcock, Frank and D. J. Mosely. *Diplomacy in Ancient Greece*. New York: St. Martin's Press, 1975.

Adshead, S.A.M. *China in World History*. New York: St. Martin's Press, 1988.

Allen, Charles, ed., with Michael Mason. *Tales from the South China Seas: Images of the British in South-East Asia in the Twentieth Century*. London: Futura Publications, 1990.

Alperovitz, Gar. *The Decision to Use the Atomic Bomb and the Architecture of an American Myth*. New York: Alfred A. Knopf, 1995.

Ambrose, Stephen E. *Nixon, Vol. 2: The Triumph of a Politician, 1962–1972*. New York: Simon & Schuster, 1989.

American Civil Liberties Union. *Civil Liberties in America: A Special Two-Year Report on the ACLU's Defense of the Bill of Rights against the Attacks of the Administration and Its Allies*. New York: American Civil Liberties Union, October 1982.

Anderson, E. N. *The Food of China*. New Haven, Conn. and London: Yale University Press, 1988.

Anderson, George L., ed. *Issues and Conflicts*. Lawrence: University of Kansas Press, 1959.

Anderson, M. S. *The Rise of Modern Diplomacy, 1450–1919*. London: Longman, 1993.

Andrews, Allen. *The Royal Whore: Barbara Villiers, Countess of Castlemaine*. Philadelphia: Chilton Book Co., 1970.

Angold, Michael. *The Byzantine Empire 1025–1204: A Political History*. London and New York: Longman, 1984.

Asprey, Robert B. *War in the Shadows: The Guerrilla in History, Vol. 1*. Garden City, N.Y.: Doubleday & Co., 1975.

Athenaeus. *The Deipnosophists, Vol. 5*, trans. Charles Burton Gulick. Cambridge, Mass.: Harvard University Press; London: Heinemann, 1933.

Atwood, Rodney. *The Hessians: Mercenaries from Hessen-Kassel in the American Revolution*. Cambridge: Cambridge University Press, 1980.

Ballhatchet, Kenneth. *Race, Sex, and Class under the Raj: Imperial Attitudes and Policies and Their Critics, 1793–1905*. New York: St. Martin's Press, 1980.

Balsdon, J.V.D.P. *Romans and Aliens*. Chapel Hill: University of North Carolina Press, 1979.

Barber, Peter. *Diplomacy: The World of the Honest Spy*. London: The British Library, 1979.

Bemis, Samuel Flagg. *Pinckney's Treaty: America's Advantage from Europe's Distress, 1783–1800*, rev. ed. New Haven, Conn.: Yale University Press, 1960.

Beringer, Richard E., Herman Hattaway, Archer Jones, and William N. Still, Jr. *Why the South Lost the Civil War*. Athens: University of Georgia Press, 1986.

Bidwell, Shelford. *Swords for Hire: European Mercenaries in Eighteenth-Century India*. London: John Murray, 1971.

Billias, George Athan. *Elbridge Gerry: Founding Father and Republican Statesman*. New York: McGraw-Hill, 1976.

Birely, Robert. *The Counter-Reformation Prince: Anti-Machiavellianism or Catholic Statecraft in Early Modern Europe*. Chapel Hill: University of North Carolina Press, 1990.

Bouwsma, William J. *Venice and the Defense of Republican Liberty: Renaissance Values in the Age of the Counter Reformation*. Berkeley: University of California Press, 1968.

Boyd, Steven R., ed. *The Whiskey Rebellion: Past and Present Perspectives*. Westport, Conn.: Greenwood Press, 1985.

Brand, Charles M. *Byzantium Confronts the West 1180–1204*. Cambridge, Mass.: Harvard University Press, 1968.

Brauchli, Marcus W. "Asians Strive to Get in the Picture with Bill: Clinton Photos, Inaugural Tickets Form Symbols of Power." *Wall Street Journal*, December 27, 1996, p. A4.

Brehier, Louis. *The Life and Death of Byzantium*, trans. Margaret Vaughan. Amsterdam: North-Holland, 1977.

Breslin, Thomas A. *China, American Catholicism, and the Missionary*. University Park: Pennsylvania State University Press, 1980.

———. "Mystifying the Past: Establishment Historians and the Origins of the Pacific War." *Bulletin of Concerned Asian Scholars* 8:4 (October–December 1976), pp. 18–36.

Bunge, William. *Nuclear War Atlas*. Oxford: Basil Blackwell, 1988.

Bunyan, Tony. *The History and Practice of the Political Police in England*. London: Quartet, 1977.

Burch, Philip H., Jr. *Elites in American History, Vol. 2: The Civil War to the New Deal.* New York: Holmes and Meier, 1981.

Burn, Andrew Robert. *Persia and the Greeks: The Defence of the West, c. 546–478 B.C.* London: Edward Arnold, 1962.

Caesar, Caius Julius. *The Gallic War,* trans. H. J. Edwards. Cambridge, Mass.: Harvard University Press; London: W. Heinemann, 1917.

Center for Defense Information. *The Defense Monitor* 24:3 (1995).

———. *The Defense Monitor* 25:4 (1996), p. 6.

———. *The Defense Monitor* 28:2 (1999), pp. 3–4.

Challener, Richard D. *Admirals, Generals, and American Foreign Policy, 1898–1914.* Princeton, N.J.: Princeton University Press, 1973.

Chang, K. C., ed. *Food in Chinese Culture: Anthropological and Historical Perspectives.* New Haven, Conn.: Yale University Press, 1977.

Charlesworth, M. P. *Trade-Routes and Commerce of the Roman Empire,* 2nd rev. ed. Chicago: Ares, 1974.

Cicero, Marcus Tullius. *De Senectute, De Amicitia, De Divinatione,* trans. William Armistead Falconer. Cambridge, Mass.: Harvard University Press; London: W. Heinemann, 1923.

Colley, Linda. *Britons: Forging the Nation 1707–1837.* New Haven, Conn. and London: Yale University Press, 1992.

Collin, Richard H. "New Directions in the Foreign Relations Historiography of Theodore Roosevelt and William Howard Taft." *Diplomatic History* 19:3 (Summer 1995), pp. 473–497.

Combs, Jerald A. *The Jay Treaty: Political Battleground of the Founding Fathers.* Berkeley: University of California Press, 1970.

Costello, John. *Virtue under Fire: How World War II Changed Our Social and Sexual Attitudes.* Boston: Little, Brown and Co., 1985.

Costigliola, Frank. " 'Unceasing Pressure for Penetration': Gender, Pathology, and Emotion in George Kennan's Formation of the Cold War." *Journal of American History* 83:4 (March 1997), pp. 1309–1339.

Cox, Allan J. *Confessions of a Corporate Headhunter.* New York: Trident Press, 1973.

Crane, Daniel M. and Thomas A. Breslin. *An Ordinary Relationship: American Opposition to Republican Revolution in China.* Miami: Florida International University Press, 1986.

Cray, Ed. *General of the Army: George C. Marshall, Soldier and Statesman.* New York: W. W. Norton & Co., 1990.

Crosby, Alfred W. *Germs, Seeds, & Animals: Studies in Ecological History.* Armonk, N.Y.: M. E. Sharpe, 1994.

Crowl, Philip A. "Forestal, James Vincent." In *Dictionary of American Biography,* Supplement Four, 1946–1950. New York: Charles Scribner's Sons, 1974.

D'Arms, John H. *Commerce and Social Standing in Ancient Rome.* Cambridge, Mass.: Harvard University Press, 1981.

Davidson, James N. *Courtesans & Fishcakes: The Consuming Passions of Classical Athens.* New York: St. Martin's Press, 1998.

de Callieres, Francois. *On the Manner of Negotiating with Princes; on the Uses of*

Diplomacy; the Choice of Ministers and Envoys; and the Personal Qualities Necessary for Success Abroad, trans. A. F. Whyte. Notre Dame, Ind.: University of Notre Dame Press, 1963 (orig. pub. Paris, 1716).

de Keijzer, Arne J. with the collaboration of Allan H. Lu. *China: Business Strategies for the '90s.* Berkeley, Calif.: Pacific View Press, 1992.

de Mause, Lloyd. *Reagan's America.* New York: Creative Roots, 1984.

Dennis, George T., trans. *Three Byzantine Military Treatises.* Washington, D.C.: Dumbarton Oaks Research Library and Collection, 1985.

de Paor, Liam. *The Peoples of Ireland: From Prehistory to Modern Times.* London: Hutchinson; Notre Dame, Ind.: University of Notre Dame Press, 1986.

Despres, John, Lilita Dzirkals, and Barton Whaley. *Timely Lessons of History: The Manchurian Model for Soviet Strategy.* A report prepared for the Office of the Secretary of Defense/Director of Net Assessment. Santa Monica, Calif.: RAND Corporation, R-1825-NA, July 1976.

Desruisseaux, Paul. "U.S. Is Less Hospitable Nowadays, Foreign Students and Scholars Find." *The Chronicle of Higher Education,* November 29, 1996, p. A45.

Diehl, Charles. *Byzantium: Greatness and Decline,* trans. Naomi Walford. New Brunswick, N.J.: Rutgers University Press, 1957.

Dillon, Wilton. *Gifts and Nations: The Obligation to Give, Receive and Repay.* The Hague: Mouton, 1968.

Dio Cocceianus, Casseius. *Dio's Roman History, Vol. 8,* with an English translation by Earnest Cary, Ph.D., on the basis of the version of Herbert Baldwin Foster. Cambridge, Mass.: Harvard University Press; London: W. Heinemann, 1925.

Dower, John W. *Japan in War and Peace: Selected Essays.* New York: New Press, 1993.

Drexler, Robert W. *Guilty of Making Peace: A Biography of Nicholas P. Trist.* Lanham, Md.: University Press of America, 1991.

Dugger, Ronnie. *On Reagan: The Man and His Presidency.* New York: McGraw-Hill, 1983.

Dvornik, Francis. *Origins of Intelligence Services: The Ancient Near East, Persia, Greece, Rome, Byzantium, the Arab Muslim Empires, the Mongol Empire, China, Muscovy.* New Brunswick, N.J.: Rutgers University Press, 1974.

Dyson, Stephen L. *The Creation of the Roman Frontier.* Princeton, N.J.: Princeton University Press, 1985.

Eisenberg, Carolyn Woods. *Drawing the Line: The American Decision to Divide Germany, 1944–1949.* Cambridge: Cambridge University Press, 1996.

Ellis, Peter Berresford. *Hell or Connaught! The Cromwellian Colonization of Ireland 1652–1660.* New York: St. Martin's Press, 1975.

Feigon, Lee. *Demystifying Tibet: Unlocking the Secrets of the Land of the Snows.* Chicago: Ivan R. Dee, 1996.

Feis, Herbert. *Three International Episodes Seen from E. A.* New York: W. W. Norton & Co., 1966.

Ferrell, Robert H. *American Diplomacy: A History.* New York: W. W. Norton & Co., 1969.

Fiedler, Tom. "Protecting Clinton Took Planning, Skill, and Lots of People." *Miami Herald*, December 12, 1994, p. 17A.

Fischer, David Hackett. *Albion's Seed: Four British Folkways in America*. New York: Oxford University Press, 1989.

Foner, Philip S. *The Spanish-Cuban-American War and the Birth of American Imperialism, Vol. 2: 1898–1902*. New York: Monthly Review Press, 1972.

Ford, Henry Jones. *The Scotch-Irish in America*. Princeton, N.J.: Princeton University Press, 1915; reprint, Hamden, Conn.: Archon Books, 1966.

Foreign Broadcast Information Service. *China Report*, July 19, 1996, p. 80.

Fry, Michael G. *Lloyd George and Foreign Policy: Vol. 1, The Education of a Statesman: 1890–1916*. Montreal: McGill–Queen's University Press, 1977.

Gaiter, Dorothy G. and John Brecher. "Tastings: Secrets of the White House Wine List." *Wall Street Journal*, June 5, 1998, p. W3.

Garnsey, Peter and Richard Saller. *The Roman Empire: Economy, Society, and Culture*. Berkeley: University of California Press, 1987.

Geanakoplos, Deno John. *Byzantium: Church, Society, and Civilization Seen through Contemporary Eyes*. Chicago: University of Chicago Press, 1984.

Gipson, Lawrence Henry. *The British Isles and the American Colonies: Great Britain and Ireland 1748–1754*. New York: Alfred A. Knopf, 1966.

Gladney, Dru C. "Representing Nationality in China: Refiguring Majority/Minority Identities." *The Journal of Asian Studies* 53:1 (February 1994), pp. 92–123.

Goeldenboog, Christian. "The Fulbright Program: Promoting Understanding." *Deutschland: Magazine on Politics, Culture, Business and Science* no. 6 (December 1995), pp. 28–31.

Gould, Jay M. with members of the Radiation and Public Health Project, Ernest J. Sternglass, Joseph Mangano, and William McDonnell. *The Enemy Within: The High Cost of Living Near Nuclear Reactors: Breast Cancer, Low Birthweights, and Other Radiation-Induced Immune Deficiency Effects*. New York: Four Walls Eight Windows, 1996.

Graber, D. A. *Crisis Diplomacy: A History of U.S. Intervention Policies and Practices*. Washington, D.C.: Public Affairs Press, 1959.

Graham, Gerald S. *Great Britain in the Indian Ocean: A Study of Maritime Enterprise, 1810–1850*. Oxford: Clarendon Press, 1967.

Green, Charles. "Fees OK for Lawmakers to Pocket Could Land Others in Jail." *Miami Herald*, September 4, 1989, p. 13A.

Greenberger, Robert S. "Foreigners Use Bribes to Beat U.S. Rivals in Many Deals, New Report Concludes." *Wall Street Journal*, October 12, 1995, p. A3.

———. "Let Me In: Taiwan, Trying to Win Status in Washington, Targets Grass Roots." *Wall Street Journal*, May 6, 1995, p. A1.

Greenstein, Fred I. *The Hidden-Hand Presidency: Eisenhower as Leader*. New York: Basic Books, 1982.

Griffiths, Percival. *The British Impact on India*. Hamden, Conn.: Archon Books, 1965.

Guerdan, Rene. *Byzantium: Its Triumphs and Tragedy*, trans. D.L.B. Hartley, with a preface by Charles Diehl. New York: G. P. Putnam's Sons, 1957.

Gulick, Edward Vose. *Europe's Classical Balance of Power: A Case History of the*

Theory and Practice of One of the Great Concepts of European Statecraft. New York: Norton, 1955.

Haggie, Paul. *Britannia at Bay: The Defence of the British Empire against Japan, 1931–1941*. Oxford: Clarendon Press, 1981.

Hale, J. R. *Florence and the Medici: The Pattern of Control*. London: Thames and Hudson, 1977.

Hall, Peter Dobkin. *The Organization of American Culture, 1700–1900: Private Institutions, Elites, and the Origins of American Nationality*. New York: New York University Press, 1984.

Halliday, Jon. *A Political History of Japanese Capitalism*. New York: Random House, 1975.

Harris, Lillian Craig. "Xinjiang, Central Asia and the Implications for China's Policy in the Islamic World." *China Quarterly* 33 (March 1993), pp. 111–129.

Harrop, William C. "The Infrastructure of American Diplomacy." *American Diplomacy* 5:3 (Summer 2000). http://www.unc.edu/depts/diplomat/AD_Issues/amdipl_16/harrop_rand1.html.

Haussig, H. W. *A History of Byzantine Civilization*, trans. J. M. Hussey. New York: Praeger, 1971.

Hayashi, Saburo in collaboration with Alvin D. Coox. *Kogun: The Japanese Army in the Pacific War*. Quantico, Va.: The Marine Corps Association, 1959.

Heald, Morrell and Lawrence S. Kaplan. *Culture and Diplomacy: The American Experience*. Westport, Conn.: Greenwood Press, 1977.

Hein, Laura. "Remembering the Bomb: The Fiftieth Anniversary in the United States and Japan. Introduction: The Bomb as Public History and Transnational Memory." *Bulletin of Concerned Asian Scholars* 27:2 (April–June 1995), pp. 3–15.

Hibbert, Christopher. *Venice: The Biography of a City*. New York: W. W. Norton & Co., 1989.

Hinsley F. H., ed. *British Foreign Policy under Sir Edward Grey*. Cambridge: Cambridge University Press, 1977.

Hitchens, Christopher. *Blood, Class, and Nostalgia: Anglo-American Ironies*. New York: Farrar, Straus & Giroux, 1990.

Hixson, Walter L. *George F. Kennan: Cold War Iconoclast*. New York: Columbia University Press, 1989.

Holmes, T. Rice. *The Architect of the Roman Empire*. Oxford: Clarendon Press, 1928; reprint, New York: AMS Press, 1977.

Hoogenboom, Ari. *Rutherford B. Hayes: Warrior and President*. Lawrence: University Press of Kansas, 1995.

Hopwood, Derek. *Sexual Encounters in the Middle East: The British, the French and the Arabs*. Reading, England: Ithaca Press, 1999.

Hunt, Albert R. "More Foreign Aid, but Less for Israel." *Wall Street Journal*, March 27, 1997, p. A23.

Hunt, Alfred N. *Haiti's Influence on Antebellum America: Slumbering Volcano in the Caribbean*. Baton Rouge: Louisiana State University Press, 1988.

Hyam, Ronald. "Empire and Sexual Opportunity." *The Journal of Imperial and Commonwealth History* 14 (January 1986), pp. 34–90.

――――. *Empire and Sexuality: The British Experience*. Manchester, England: Manchester University Press; New York: St. Martin's Press, 1990.

Ienaga, Saburo. *The Pacific War, 1931–1945: A Critical Perspective on Japan's Role in World War II*. New York: Pantheon Books, 1978.

Ignatiev, Noel. *How the Irish Became White*. New York: Routledge, 1995.

Ireye, Akira. *From Nationalism to Internationalism: US Foreign Policy to 1914*. London: Henley; Boston: Routledge & Kegan Paul, 1977.

Jagchid, Sechin and Van Jay Symons. *Peace, War, and Trade along the Great Wall: Nomadic-Chinese Interaction through Two Millennia*. Bloomington: Indiana University Press, 1989.

Jensen, Ronald J. *The Alaska Purchase and Russian–American Relations*. Seattle and London: University of Washington Press, 1975.

Johnson, Haynes and Bernard M. Gwertzman. *Fulbright: The Dissenter*. Garden City, N.Y.: Doubleday & Co., 1968.

Johnston, Alastair Iain. *Cultural Realism: Strategic Culture and Grand Strategy in Chinese History*. Princeton, N.J.: Princeton University Press, 1995.

Kaegi, Walter Emil, Jr. *Byzantine Military Unrest, 471–843: An Interpretation*. Amsterdam: Walter M. Hakkert, 1981.

Kapelle, William E. *The Norman Conquest of the North: The Region and Its Transformation, 1000–1135*. Chapel Hill: University of North Carolina Press, 1979.

Kaplan, David E. *Fires of the Dragon: Politics, Murder, and the Kuomintang*. New York: Atheneum, 1992.

Kaplan, David E. and Alec Dubro. *Yakuza: The Explosive Account of Japan's Criminal Underworld*. Reading, Mass.: Addison-Wesley, 1986.

Kaplan, Lawrence S. *Colonies into Nation: American Diplomacy, 1763–1801*. New York: Macmillan, 1972.

Kazuo, Ogura. "How the 'Inscrutables' Negotiate with the 'Inscrutables': Chinese Negotiating Tactics vis-à-vis the Japanese." *China Quarterly* 79 (September 1979), pp. 529–552.

Keatley, Robert. "U.S. Campaign against Bribery Faces Resistance from Foreign Governments." *Wall Street Journal*, February 4, 1994, p. A4.

Kellerman, Henry J. *Cultural Relations as an Instrument of U.S. Foreign Policy: The Educational Exchange Program between the United States and Germany, 1945–1954*. Department of State Publication 8931: International Information and Cultural Series 114. Washington, D.C.: U.S. Government Printing Office, 1978.

Kennan, George F. *Soviet-American Relations, 1917–1920, Vol. 2: The Decision to Intervene*. Princeton, N.J.: Princeton University Press, 1958.

King, Neil, Jr. "Bribery Ban Is Approved by OECD." *Wall Street Journal*, November 24, 1997, p. A14.

Kissinger, Henry. *White House Years*. Boston: Little, Brown and Co., 1979.

Kofsky, Frank. *Harry S. Truman and the War Scare of 1948: A Successful Campaign to Deceive the Nation*. New York: St. Martin's Press, 1993.

――――. "Truman, Byrnes and the Atomic Bomb." *Newsletter of the Society for Historians of American Foreign Relations* 27:2 (June 1996), pp. 16–30.

Kolko, Gabriel. *The Politics of War: The World and United States Foreign Policy, 1943–1945.* New York: Random House, 1970.

Kotschevar, Lendel H. "French and Chinese Cuisines: An Evaluation." *FIU Hospitality Review* 3:1 (Spring 1985), pp. 25–34.

Kunz, Diane B. "When Money Counts and Doesn't: Economic Power and Diplomatic Objectives." *Diplomatic History* 18:4 (Fall 1994), pp. 451–462.

Lane, Frederic C. *Venice: A Maritime Republic.* Baltimore: Johns Hopkins University Press, 1973.

Lattimore, Owen. *Inner Asian Frontiers of China,* 2nd ed. Irvington-on-Hudson, N.Y.: Capitol Publishing Co.; New York: American Geographical Society, 1951.

Lauritzen, Peter. *Venice: A Thousand Years of Culture and Civilization.* New York: Atheneum, 1978.

Leung, Julia. "Greased Palms Lubricate Wheels in China: Foreign Businessmen Find Everyone's Looking to Be Paid Off." *Wall Street Journal,* July 20, 1989, p. A10.

Lewis, Gordon K. *Slavery, Imperialism, and Freedom: Essays in English Radical Thought.* New York: Monthly Review Press, 1968.

Liggio, Leonard P. and James J. Martin, eds. *Watershed of Empire: Essays on New Deal Foreign Policy.* Colorado Springs: Ralph Myles, 1976.

"London Broil Follows Press Sex Expose." *Miami Herald,* March 19, 1989, p. 3A.

Lopez, Claude-Anne. *Mon Cher Papa: Franklin and the Ladies of Paris.* New Haven, Conn.: Yale University Press, 1967.

Lowe, C. J. *The Reluctant Imperialists: British Foreign Policy 1878–1902.* New York: Macmillan, 1969.

Luan, Baoqun, comp. *Tales from the Imperial Palace of Anicent China, Vol. 1: Tales About Chinese Emperors—Their Wild and Wise Ways.* Hong Kong: Hai Feng Publishing Co., 1994.

Luttwak, Edward N. *The Grand Strategy of the Roman Empire from the First Century A.D. to the Third.* Baltimore: Johns Hopkins University Press, 1976.

Machiavelli, Niccolò. *The Portable Machiavelli,* trans. and ed. with a critical introduction by Peter Bondanella and Mark Musa. New York: Penguin Books, 1979.

———. *The Prince,* trans. and ed. Robert M. Adams. New York: W. W. Norton & Co., 1977.

MacMullen, Ramsay. *Corruption and the Decline of Rome.* New Haven, Conn. and London: Yale University Press, 1988.

———. *Enemies of the Roman Order: Treason, Unrest, and Alienation in the Empire.* Cambridge, Mass.: Harvard University Press, 1966.

McGregor, James. "The Opium War: Burma Road Heroin Breeds Addicts, AIDS along China's Border." *Wall Street Journal,* September 29, 1992, p. A1.

———. "Taiwan Cultivates America's Support with Lobbying Force the Size of Israel's." *Wall Street Journal,* January 7, 1989, p. A26.

McLaren, Anne E., trans. and ed. *The Chinese Femme Fatale: Stories from the Ming Period.* Sydney: Wild Peony, 1994.

McMurry, Ruth Emily and Muna Lee. *The Cultural Approach: Another Way in*

International Relations. Chapel Hill: University of North Carolina Press, 1947; reprint, Port Washington, N.Y.: Kennikat Press, 1972.

McWhiney, Grady. *Cracker Culture: Celtic Ways in the Old South*. Tuscaloosa: University of Alabama Press, 1988.

Mahoney, Rosemary. *The Early Arrival of Dreams: A Year in China*. New York: Fawcett Columbine, 1990; paperback ed., 1992.

Mancall, Peter C. *Deadly Medicine: Indians and Alcohol in Early America*. Ithaca, N.Y.: Cornell University Press, 1995.

———. *Valley of Opportunity: Economic Culture along the Upper Susquehanna, 1700–1800*. Ithaca, N.Y.: Cornell University Press, 1991.

Mansourov, Alexandre Y. "Stalin, Mao, Kim, and China's Decision to Enter the Korean War, September 16–October 15, 1950: New Evidence from the Russian Archives." The Cold War International History Project *Bulletin*, issues 6–7 (Winter 1995–1996). Washington, D.C.: Woodrow Wilson International Center for Scholars, pp. 94–119.

Marshall, Jonathan. "The Institute of Pacific Relations: Politics and Polemics." *Bulletin of Concerned Asian Scholars* 8:2 (April–June 1976), pp. 35–44.

———. "Opium and the Politics of Gangsterism in Nationalist China, 1927–1945." *Bulletin of Concerned Asian Scholars* 8:3 (July–September 1976), pp. 19–48.

———. *To Have and Have Not: Southeast Asian Raw Materials and the Origins of the Pacific War*. Berkeley: University of California Press, 1995.

Matthewson, Timothy M. "George Washington's Policy toward the Haitian Revolution." *Diplomatic History* 3:3 (Summer 1979), pp. 321–336.

Maurois, Andre. *Chateaubriand: Poet, Statesman, Lover*, trans. Vera Fraser. New York: Greenwood Press, 1969 (orig. pub. 1938).

May, Glenn Anthony. *Social Engineering in the Philippines: The Aims, Execution, and Impact of American Colonial Policy, 1900–1913*. Westport, Conn.: Greenwood Press, 1980.

Mead, Walter Russell. "The Two Trillion Dollar Mistake." *Worth* 5:2 (February 1996), p. 76.

Middleton, Charles Ronald. *The Administration of British Foreign Policy 1782–1846*. Durham, N.C.: Duke University Press, 1977.

Mintz, Sidney W. *Sweetness and Power: The Place of Sugar in Modern History*. New York: Viking, 1985.

Moon, Penderel. *The British Conquest and Dominion of India*. London: Duckworth, 1989.

Mosher, Steven W. *China Misperceived: American Illusions and Chinese Reality*. New York: Basic Books, 1990.

Murphey, Rhoads. *The Outsiders: The Western Experience in India and China*. Ann Arbor: University of Michigan Press, 1977.

Nichols, Kenneth. *Gaelic and Gaelicized Ireland in the Middle Ages*. Dublin: Gill and MacMillan, 1972.

O'Brien, Michael J. *A Hidden Phase of American History: Ireland's Part in America's Struggle for Liberty*. N.p., 1919; reprint, Freeport, N.Y.: Books for Libraries Press, 1971.

Olmstead, A. T. *History of the Persian Empire*. Chicago: University of Chicago Press, 1948 (6th ed., 1970).

Ostrogorsky, George. *History of the Byzantine State*, rev. ed., trans. Joan Hussey, with a foreword by Peter Charanis. New Brunswick, N.J.: Rutgers University Press, 1969.

Pach, Chester J., Jr. and Elmo Richardson. *The Presidency of Dwight D. Eisenhower*, rev. ed. Lawrence: University Press of Kansas, 1991.

Paolino, Ernest N. *The Foundations of the American Empire: William Henry Seward and U.S. Foreign Policy*. Ithaca, N.Y. and London: Cornell University Press, 1973.

Parker, R.A.C. *Chamberlain and Appeasement: British Policy and the Coming of the Second World War*. New York: St. Martin's Press, 1993.

Paterson, Thomas G., J. Gary Clifford, and Kenneth J. Hagan. *American Foreign Relations: A History to 1920*, 4th ed. Lexington, Mass.: D. C. Heath and Co., 1995.

Phillips, Michael. "Chinese Government Paid for Shaw's Trip." *Miami Herald*, November 29, 1990, p. 16A.

Pisani, Sallie. *The CIA and the Marshall Plan*. Lawrence: University Press of Kansas, 1991.

Platt, D.C.M. *The Cinderella Service: British Consuls since 1825*. London: Longman, 1971.

Plutarch. "Pericles." In *The Lives of the Noble Grecians and Romans*, trans. John Dryden, rev. Arthur Hugh Clough. New York: Modern Library, n.d.

Powers, Thomas. *Heisenberg's War: The Secret History of the German Bomb*. Boston: Little, Brown and Co., 1993.

Preston, William, Jr., Edward S. Herman, and Herbert I. Schiller. *Hope & Folly: The United States and UNESCO, 1945–1985*. Minneapolis: University of Minnesota Press, 1989.

Propas, Frederic L. "Creating a Hard Line toward Russia: The Training of State Department Soviet Experts, 1927–1937." *Diplomatic History* 8:3 (Summer 1984), pp. 209–226.

Prucha, Francis Paul. *The Great Father: The United States Government and the American Indians, Vol. 1*. Lincoln: University of Nebraska Press, 1984.

Queller, Donald E. *The Office of Ambassador in the Middle Ages*. Princeton, N.J.: Princeton University Press, 1967.

Quinn, David Beers. *The Elizabethans and the Irish*. Ithaca, N.Y.: Cornell University Press, 1966.

Reid, John Phillip. *In a Defiant Stance: The Conditions of Law in Massachusetts Bay, the Irish Comparison, and the Coming of the American Revolution*. University Park: Pennsylvania State University Press, 1977.

Riding, Alan. "Brazil Gives Jimmy Carter a Warm Welcome." *New York Times*, October 9, 1984, p. 4.

Robertson, David. *Sly and Able: A Political Biography of James F. Byrnes*. New York: W. W. Norton & Co., 1994.

Rocca, Jean-Louis. "Corruption and Its Shadow: An Anthropological View of Corruption in China." *China Quarterly* 130 (June 1992), pp. 402–416.

Roeber, A. G. *Palatines, Liberty, and Property: German Lutherans in Colonial British America*. Baltimore: Johns Hopkins University Press, 1993.

Rosenthal, Andrew. "The Raising of Funds: Lessons in Superpower Reciprocity." *New York Times*, August 25, 1987, p. 10.

Rosenthal, Margaret F. *The Honest Courtesan: Veronica Franco, Citizen and Writer in Sixteenth-Century Venice*. Chicago: University of Chicago Press, 1992.

Rossabi, Morris. *China and Inner Asia: From 1368 to the Present Day*. New York: Pica Press, 1975.

Rossabi, Morris, ed. *China among Equals: The Middle Kingdom and Its Neighbors, 10th–14th Centuries*. Berkeley: University of California Press, 1983.

Rotberg, Robert I. with the collaboration of Miles F. Shore. *The Founder: Cecil Rhodes and the Pursuit of Power*. New York: Oxford University Press, 1988.

Rowdon, Maurice. *The Silver Age of Venice*. New York: Praeger, 1970.

Rubin, Amy Magaro. "Fulbright Program Adjusts to a Smaller Fellowship Budget." *The Chronicle of Higher Education*, May 31, 1996, p. A34.

———. "Fulbright Program Fights to Stay Alive in Face of Severe Cuts." *The Chronicle of Higher Education*, March 15, 1996, p. A45.

Sale, Kirkpatrick. *Power Shift: The Rise of the Southern Rim and Its Challenge to the Eastern Establishment*. New York: Random House, 1975.

Sanders, Jerry W. *Peddlers of Crisis: The Committee on the Present Danger and the Politics of Containment*. Boston: South End Press, 1983.

Schafer, Edward H. *The Golden Peaches of Samarkand: A Study in T'ang Exotics*. Berkeley: University of California Press, 1963.

Schaller, Michael. *The American Occupation of Japan: The Origins of the Cold War in Asia*. New York: Oxford University Press, 1985.

Schevill, Ferdinand. *History of Florence, from the Founding of the City through the Renaissance*. New York: Frederick Ungar, 1968.

Schroeder, Paul. "Historical Reality vs. Neo-Realist Theory." *International Security* 19:1 (Summer 1994), pp. 108–148.

Schwenninger, Sherle R. "The Debate That Wasn't: Foreign Policy Questions Were Not-So-Curiously Absent from the Campaign Trail." *The Nation* 263:16 (November 18, 1996), pp. 22–24.

Scott, H. M. *British Foreign Policy in the Age of the American Revolution*. Oxford: Clarendon Press, 1990.

Scott, Peter Dale. *Deep Politics and the Death of JFK*. Berkeley: University of California Press, 1993.

Seagrave, Sterling. *The Soong Dynasty*. New York: Harper & Row, 1985.

Searle, G. R. *Entrepreneurial Politics in Mid-Victorian Britain*. Oxford: Oxford University Press, 1993.

Shakabpa, Tsepon W. D. *Tibet: A Political History*. New Haven, Conn.: Yale University Press, 1967.

Sheehan, Bernard W. *Seeds of Extinction: Jeffersonian Philanthropy and the American Indian*. Chapel Hill: University of North Carolina Press for the Institute of Early American History and Culture at Williamsburg, Virginia, 1973.

Sheridan, Mary Beth. "The Spirit of Miami." *Miami Herald*, December 12, 1994, p. 1A.

Sherry, Michael S. *In the Shadow of War: The United States since the 1930s*. New Haven, Conn.: Yale University Press, 1995.

Sherwig, John M. *Guineas and Gunpowder: British Foreign Aid in the Wars with France, 1793–1815*. Cambridge, Mass.: Harvard University Press, 1969.

Shibama, C., comp. *The First Japanese Embassy to the United States of America: Sent to Washington as the First of the Series of Embassies Specially Sent Abroad by the Tokugawa Shogunate*. Tokyo: The America–Japan Society, 1920.

Shoup, Laurence H. and William Minter. *Imperial Brain Trust: The Council on Foreign Relations and United States Foreign Policy*. New York: Monthly Review Press, 1977.

Slevin, Peter. "Foreign Aid, Diplomacy Hit Hard by Cuts." *Miami Herald*, May 5, 1996, p. 18A.

Smith, George Winston and Charles Judah, eds. *Chronicles of the Gringos: The U.S. Army in the Mexican War, 1846–1848, Accounts of Eyewitnesses and Combatants*. Albuquerque: University of New Mexico Press, 1968.

Socolofsky, Homer E. and Allan B. Spetter. *The Presidency of Benjamin Harrison*. Lawrence: University Press of Kansas, 1987.

Sofka, James R. "The Jeffersonian Idea of National Security: Commerce, the Atlantic Balance of Power, and the Barbary War, 1786–1805." *Diplomatic History* 21:4 (Fall 1997), pp. 519–544.

Spiele, Hilde, ed. *The Congress of Vienna: An Eyewitness Account*, trans. Richard H. Weber. Philadelphia: Chilton Book Co., 1968.

Starr, Chester G. *The Roman Empire 27 B.C.–A.D. 476: A Study in Survival*. New York: Oxford University Press, 1982.

Stephanson, Anders. *Manifest Destiny: American Expansionism and the Empire of Right*. New York: Hill and Wang, 1995.

Stettinius, Edward R., Jr. *Lend-Lease: Weapon for Victory*. New York: Macmillan, 1944.

Stevenson, Richard W. "Ex-Bomb Designer Wins Peace Prize: He Quit Manhattan Project and Led Anti-Nuclear Campaign." *Miami Herald*, October 14, 1995, p. 1A.

Stockwell, John. *The Praetorian Guard: The U.S. Role in the New World Order*. Boston: South End Press, 1991.

Stross, Randall E. *Bulls in the China Shop and Other Sino-American Business Encounters*. New York: Pantheon, 1991.

Sun, Haichen, comp. and trans. *The Wiles of War: 36 Military Strategies from Ancient China*. Beijing: Foreign Languages Press, 1991.

Tansill, Charles C. *The Foreign Policy of Thomas F. Bayard, 1885–1897*. New York: Fordham University Press, 1940; reprint, New York: Kraus Reprint Co., 1969.

Tao, Hanzhang. *Sun Tzu's Art of War: The Modern Chinese Interpretation*, trans. Yuan Shibing. New York: Sterling Publishing Co., 1987.

Tao, Jing-shen. *The Jurchen in Twelfth-Century China: A Study of Sinicization*. Seattle: University of Washington Press, 1976.

Taylor, A.J.P. *English History 1914–1945*. Oxford and New York: Oxford University Press, 1965.

Theoharis, Athan. *Seeds of Repression: Harry S. Truman and the Origins of McCarthyism*. Chicago: Quadrangle Books, 1971.

Thompson, James Westfall and Saul K. Padover. *Secret Diplomacy: Espionage and Cryptography, 1500–1815*, 2nd ed. New York: Frederick Ungar, 1963. (Originally published as *Secret Diplomacy, A Record of Espionage and Double-Dealing: 1500–1815*. London: Jarrolds, 1937.)

Thucydides. *History of the Peloponnesian War*, trans. Charles Forster Smith. Cambridge, Mass.: Harvard University Press; London: W. Heinemann, 1919.

Timperlake, Edward and William C. Triplett II. *Year of the Rat: How Bill Clinton Compromised U.S. Security for Cash*. Washington, D.C.: Regnery Publishing Co., 1998.

Toynbee, Arnold. *Constantine Porphyrogenitus and His World*. London: Oxford University Press, 1973.

Trento, Susan B. *The Power House: Robert Keith Gray and the Selling of Access and Influence in Washington*. New York: St. Martin's Press, 1992.

Tucker, Robert W. and David C. Hendrickson. *The Fall of the First British Empire: Origins of the War of American Independence*. Baltimore and London: Johns Hopkins University Press, 1982.

Tugend, Alina. "Respected British Mathematician Takes on Nuclear-Weapons Industry." *The Chronicle of Higher Education*, April 19, 1996, p. A54.

Uhl, Michael and Tod Ensign. *G.I. Guinea Pigs: How the Pentagon Exposed Our Troops to Dangers More Deadly Than War*. N.p.: Playboy Press, dist. by Harper & Row, 1980.

Unger, Jonathan and Jean Xiong. "Life in the Chinese Hinterlands under the Rural Economic Reforms." *Bulletin of Concerned Asian Scholars* 22:2 (April–June 1990), pp. 4–17.

U.S. General Accounting Office. GAO Report B-225,870. "Foreign Aid: Improving the Impact and Control of Economic Support Funds." Report to the Chairman, Subcommittee on Europe and the Middle East, Committee on Foreign Affairs, House of Representatives, June 1988.

Valeriani, Richard. *Travels with Henry*. Boston: Houghton Mifflin, 1979.

Van Alstyne, Richard W. *Empire and Independence: The International History of the American Revolution*. New York: John Wiley & Sons, 1965.

———. *The Rising American Empire*. Oxford: Basil Blackwell, 1960.

Van Deusen, Glyndon G. *William Henry Seward*. New York: Oxford University Press, 1967.

Van Gulik, R. H. *Sexual Life in Ancient China: A Preliminary Survey of Chinese Sex and Society from ca. 1500 B.C. Till 1644 A.D.* Leiden, Netherlands: Brill, 1961; reprint, New York: Barnes & Noble Books, 1996.

Waldron, Arthur. *The Great Wall of China: From History to Myth*. Cambridge: Cambridge University Press, 1992 Canto ed.

Wang, Congren, comp. *Tales from the Imperial Palace of Ancient China, Vol. 3: Tales About Prime Ministers in Chinese History*. Hong Kong: Hai Feng Publishing Co., 1994.

Wardman, Alan. *Rome's Debt to Greece*. New York: St. Martin's Press, 1976.

Wasserman, Harvey and Norman Solomon. *Killing Our Own: The Disaster of America's Experience with Atomic Radiation.* New York: Dell Publishing Co., 1982.

Watanabe, Kazuko. "Militarism, Colonialism, and the Trafficking of Women: Comfort Women: Forced into Sexual Labor for Japanese Soldiers." *Bulletin of Concerned Asian Scholars* 26:4 (October–December 1994), pp. 3–17.

Watson, Burton, trans. *Records of the Grand Historian of China Translated from the Shih chi of Ssu-Ma Ch'ien, Vol. 2: The Age of Emperor Wu, 140 to Circa 100 B.C.* New York: Columbia University Press, 1961.

Watson, Rubie S. and Patricia Buckley Ebrey, eds. *Marriage and Inequality in Chinese Society.* Berkeley: University of California Press, 1991.

Weart, Spencer R. *Nuclear Fear: A History.* Cambridge, Mass.: Harvard University Press, 1988.

Webster, Charles. *The Congress of Vienna, 1814–1815.* New York: Barnes & Noble, 1969.

Wei, Tang. "Guan Yu: The 'God of War' Who Failed." *China Reconstructs* 32:11 (November 1983), pp. 67–68.

———. "A Kingdom Lost for a Concubine's Smile." *China Reconstructs* 31:3 (March 1982), p. 72.

———. "Wang Zhaojun: Was She Really So Sad?" *China Reconstructs* 32:7 (July 1983), pp. 65–66.

West, Richard S. *Admirals of American Empire: The Combined Story of George Dewey, Alfred Thayer Mahan, Winfield Scott Schley and William Thomas Sampson.* Indianapolis, Ind.: Bobbs-Merrill, 1948; reprint, Westport, Conn.: Greenwood Press, 1971.

Wheeler, Mortimer. *Rome beyond the Imperial Frontiers.* Westport, Conn.: Greenwood Press, 1971 (orig. pub. 1954).

"Who Needs an Army?" *The Economist,* June 4, 1994, pp. 16–18.

Wills, Garry. *Inventing America: Jefferson's Declaration of Independence.* Garden City, N.Y.: Doubleday & Co., 1978.

Winkler, John J. *The Constraints of Desire.* New York: Routledge, 1990.

Wong, Jeannie. "Institute of Peace, a Cold-War Creation, Charts New Course." *The Chronicle of Higher Education,* September 15, 1993, p. A30.

Wooldridge, Jane. "The Summit Soirees." *Miami Herald,* December 12, 1994, p. 1C.

Wooldridge, Jane, Fernando Gonzalez, and Martin Merzer. "Work's Over—Time to Boogie." *Miami Herald,* December 11, 1994, p. 39A.

Yu, Ying-shih. *Trade and Expansion in Han China: A Study in Sino-Barbarian Relations.* Berkeley: University of California Press, 1967.

Zha, Jianying. *China Pop: How Soap Operas, Tabloids, and Bestsellers Are Transforming a Culture.* New York: New Press, 1995.

Index

Adams, John, 134, 138
Adcock, Frank, 31
The Aeneid, 41
Afghanistan, 115
Africa, 49, 52, 119–20
Agislaus, Spartan King, 30–31
Agricola, 43
Alaric, Visigoth leader, 45
Alaska Purchase, 141–42, 159 nn.16, 17
Albert, Carl, 153
Alcohol. *See* Food and drink
Alexander I, Czar of Russia, 109
Alexander of Macedon, 24, 33
Alexis III, Emperor of Byzantium, 64
Alexius I Comnenus, Emperor of Byzantium, 55, 58, 68
Alliances, 3, 8, 55, 77, 93, 98, 110, 148–49, 169. *See also* Diplomacy; Marital alliances; Treaty
American Enterprise Institute, 175
American Revolution, 77, 100, 133; Hessian deserters, 96, 134; Scots and Irish as rebels, 99. *See also* United States of America
Anabasis, 30

Anderson, E. N., 171
Andronicus I, Emperor of Byzantium, 70
Andronicus II Paleologus, Emperor of Byzantium, 57
Anglo-Normans, 55, 59, 62–64, 69–70, 85, 100, 128; relations with Irish, 86–87. *See also* Britain
Angold, Michael, 54
Anna Porphyrogenita, 53
Anti-Machiavellianism, 79–80, 88
Apartheid. *See* British policy
Arabs, 11, 51–53, 59
Arms. *See* Military policy
Artabazus, rebel satrap, 32
Artaxerxes, 30
Artaxerxes III Ochus, 32
Articles of Confederation, 135–36
Artists, Venetian, 75
Aspasia, 28
Asquith, Herbert Henry, Prime Minister, 121
Athens, 23–24, 26–27; alliances, 31–32; attack on Syracuse, 29; captured, 25; treaty with Persia, 29; war with Sparta, 30

Atiyah, Michael, 126
Atomic bomb. *See* Nuclear bomb
Atwood, Rodney, 97
Austria, 74, 81, 108, 110
Avars (Uighur Turks), 50

Bagration, Princess Catherine, 109, 111
Baji Rao, Peswa of Maratha Confederation, 115
Banquets, 4, 10, 15–16, 55, 59–60, 71, 108, 157, 167. *See also* Food and drink; Hospitality
Bao, Chinese state of, 2
Barber, Peter, 90
Barry, Commodore John, 99
Basil I, Emperor of Byzantium, 51
Basil II, Emperor of Byzantium, 53–54, 65 n.10
Bayard, Thomas F., 142–43
"The Beauty Trap," 2
Belisarius, 68
Bertha of Sulzbach, 62–64
Bismarck, Otto von, 143
Black Death. *See* Plague
Boer War, 121
Bonaparte, Napoleon, 68, 77, 101, 107, 138
Bower, Captain Hamilton, 176 n.3
Brehier, Louis, 50
Bribery: by Americans, 138–39, 151; by British, 90–91, 107, 112–15, 118, 122, 135; by Byzantines, 55; by Chinese, 5–6, 12, 157, 167, 170–71, 175; by French, 77; by Greeks, 22, 26, 28, 38, 58; by Persians, 23–25, 27, 29–32; by Romans, 35, 39–40, 43, 45 n.2; by Venetians, 68–69, 72. *See also* Gift giving
Britain: attitudes about Indian women, 118, 129 n.21; behavior in America, 104 n.14; diplomatic efforts, 110–

11, 125, 135, 165; emigration to Africa, 120; policy of appeasement, 119, 123; policy of racial apartheid, 117; wartime strategy, 124; war with China, 116. *See also* American Revolution; Anglo-Normans; Civil War; French and Indian War
Brook, Charles, Second British White Rajah, 117
Bryce, James, 121
Buchanan, James, 140
Bulgaria, 51–53, 122
Burgoyne, General John, 98
Bush, George H. W., 154–55
Byroade, Henry A., Ambassador to Egypt, 151
Byzantium, 49; history, 82 nn.3, 5; relations with Arabs and Bulgars, 51–53; relations with Germans and Normans, 62–64; relations with Russia, 53; relations with Turks, 54–57; relations with Venice, 55–56, 67–68. *See also* Constantinople

Caesar, Julius, 39, 41
Callahan, Sonny, 156
Canning, George, 112, 139
Carter, James Earl, 153, 174
Castlereagh, Robert Stewart, Viscount, 111
Caulaincourt, Armand, Marquis de, 108
Celts, 35–36, 40, 43–44
Central Intelligence Agency, 151, 153
Chamberlain, Joseph: British Minister to United States of America, 143; British Prime Minister, 123, 125
Charlemagne, 58, 68
Charles III, King of Spain, 136
Charles Stuart II of Britain, 89
Chateaubriand, François-Réné, Vicomte de, 111–12

Chennault, Anna, 168
Chen Yuanyuan, concubine of Wu Sanqui, 17
China, 1; cultural assimilation, 17 n.7, 163, 168; relations with Russia, 165, 169; relations with Turks, 9–11; Second Anglo-Chinese War, 116. See also Individual dynasties and states; Khitans; Nationalist Chinese; People's Republic of China
China Lobby, 150–51, 167–68, 174
Chin dynasty, 15
Chinese National Association of Industry and Commerce, 175
Chinese People's Institute of Foreign Affairs, 171–72
Christianity. See Crusade; Religion
The Christian Politician, 80
Chu, Chinese state of, 3
Churchill, Winston, 121, 125, 128
Cicero, 38
Cimon, 26–27
Cincibilis of Noricum, 36
Citizen army. See Militia
Civil war: American, 141; British, 89
Cleopatra, 40–41
Cleveland, Grover, 142, 144
Clinton, General Sir Henry, 99
Clinton, William Jefferson, 155, 157, 174
Clive, Robert, Baron, 91
Coalition. See Alliances
Colbert de Croissy, Marqui Charles, 89
Concubine. See Women
Confederate State of America, 116
Conference of Aix-La-Chapelle, 112
Congress of Cambrai, 111
Congress of Vienna, 108–9, 128 n.9
Conrad II, German Emperor, 62
Constantine VIII, Emperor of Byzantium, 54

Constantine IX Monomachos, Emperor of Byzantium, 54
Constantinople, 40, 49, 57, 59, 71. See also Byzantium
Contzen, Adam, 80
Convention for the Promotion of Inter-American Cultural Relations, 146
Cooper, John Sherman, 151
Cooperative Threat Reduction Program, 148
Coote, Sir Eyre, 92
Corcoran, David, 166
Corcoran, Thomas G., 166
Cornwallis, General Charles, Marquis, 88, 100, 106 n.44
Council on Foreign Relations, 148
Court ceremony. See Hospitality
Courtesans. See Women
Crete, 71, 76
Crimean War, 114, 118
Cromwell, Oliver, 89
Crusade: Second, 55, 60; Fourth, 56, 70–71
Cuba, 144
Cuman, 55
Cybele, 37–38
Cyprus, 26–27, 31–32, 72, 75
Cyrus, Persian rebel, 30

DaCanale, Cristoforo, 75
Dandalo, Marco, 69
Darius II Ochus, King of Persia, 29
Darius III, King of Persia, 33
Dartmouth, William Legge, Earl of, 96
Davidson, James N., 22, 26
Davis, Jefferson, 140
Deaver, Michael, 174
Debt. See Money
de Callieres, Francois, 19 n.37, 108–10
de Commines, Philippe, 73
de Keroualle, Louise, 89
Delano, Frederick, 166

Demosthenes, 32–33

Diehl, Charles, 58

Dio Cassius, 36, 47 n.30

Diplomacy, 12–13, 15, 18 n.25, 36, 57, 64, 75, 92; enlistment of allies, 10, 50, 108, 110, 121, 133–34; study of opponents, 35, 42, 57–58; style and strategy, 8, 63, 67; use of agents, 3, 95, 109, 158 n.9; use of education, 90, 94, 144–45, 148–49, 163; use of trade and foreign aid, 9, 12, 36, 43, 151, 155, 164. *See also* Alliances; Gift giving; Hospitality; Peace; Treaty

Discourses on the First Ten Books of Titus Livius, 79

Divide and conquer strategy, 7, 11–12, 35, 50, 59, 74, 88, 120. *See also* Military strategy

Domitian, Emperor, 43

Dowry. *See* Marital alliances

Dubois, Guillaume, Cardinal, 80–81

Dulles, John Foster, 151

Dundas, Henry, Viscount Melville, 100

East India Company, 91–93, 95, 100, 129 n.21

Education for assimilation, 36, 139, 144–45, 149, 163, 175

Edward III of Britain, 77

Egypt, 27, 32, 40–41, 54, 56, 119, 151

Eirene, 52, 57–58

Eisenhower, Dwight D., 151

Ellis, Peter Berresford, 89, 102

Endicott, Mary, 143–44

Endicott, William C., 144

England. *See* Britain

Epicureans, 37

Epistles (Horace), 41

Eritrea, 23

Erskine, David, 138

Fitzgibbon, John, 102

Flattery, 38, 40, 42, 79, 101, 121, 137. *See also* Diplomacy

Florence, 67, 73–74, 77, 81

Food and drink: for Americans, 142, 144, 147, 157; for Anglo-Normans, 85; for Chinese, 1, 6, 9–10, 14, 17 n.11, 60, 171; for English, 114, 171; for French, 111; for Koreans, 14; role of supply, 27, 30–31, 54, 62, 85, 166; for Romans, 35; for Spanish, 136. *See also* Banquets; Hospitality

Ford, Henry Jones, 105 n.31

Fortifications. *See* Wall building

Fothergill, Dr. John, 94

France, 74, 80, 110–11, 121; relations with American colonies, 98, 134–35; relations with England, 87, 119, 121. *See also* French and Indian War; French Revolution

Franco, Veronica, 75, 82 n.19

Franco-American Treaty of Alliance, 138

Franco-Byzantine Treaty of 814 A.D., 68

Franke, Herbert, 18 n.25

Franklin, Benjamin, 98, 134

Franks, 68

Franz II, Emperor of Austria, 108–9

French and Indian War, 95, 133

French Revolution, 77, 101

Friendship, 22, 98, 121, 134, 146, 151, 169, 172

Fulbright Program, 149, 157

Gadsden Purchase, 140

Gage, General Thomas, 96

Gallic War, 39, 43

Galloway, Joseph, 99

Gandhi, Mahatma, 123

Gardiner, Luke, 99

Gardoqui, Diego de, 136
Gates, General Horatio, 103
Gauls. *See* Celts
Genoa, 56, 58, 70–72, 110
George I of Britain, 80
George III of Britain, 90, 93
Germain, Lord George, 99
Germania, 44
German tribes, 43–44
Germany, 62, 64, 69–70, 74, 121–25,
    143, 145–47, 156
Gift giving: by Byzantines, 58–59; by
    Chinese, 3, 7, 12–14, 16, 166–67,
    173; by English, 113, 124; by
    French, 80–81; by Germans, 145; by
    Greeks, 21, 23; by Japanese, 140; by
    Persians, 23; by Romans, 36, 38, 44;
    by Spain, 88–89, 136; by Venetians,
    74. *See also* Bribery
Gipson, Lawrence Henry, 90
Gold, 1, 56, 78–79, 111–12, 114, 138.
    See also Money; Wealth
Goths, 68, 78
Gravier, Charles Comte de Vergennes,
    135
Greece, 21, 36, 40–41, 50–51, 56–57,
    73–74, 76
Greenberger, Robert S., 175
Grenville, Lord George, 101
Guerdan, Rene, 59

Hale, J. R., 81
Hamilton, Lord George, 117
Han dynasty, 5–8
Hannaford, Peter, 174
Hartley, David, 134
Harvard University, 144–45, 150
Hastings, Governor-General Francis
    Rawdon, Marquess of, 115
Hastings, Warren, 100
Hay, John, 143
Hayes, Lucy Webb, 142
Hayes, Rutherford B., 142

Henry, Patrick, 96
Henry III, of France, 75, 82 n.19
Heqin, policy of Han, 6
Heritage Foundation, 175
Hessians, 96, 105 n.31, 134
Hinrichs, Johann, 96
The History of British India, 92
Holy Alliance, 110
Homer, 21–22
Hong Kong, 127
Hoover, J. Edgar, 152
Hopwood, Derk, 117
Horace, 41
Hospitality, 22, 40, 59, 61, 65 n.23,
    73, 81, 108, 168–70. *See also* Ban-
    quets; Food and drink
Hughes, Howard, 154
"A Hundred War Maxims," 2
Hungary, 52, 69–71
Huns, 50, 59
Hunt, Albert R., 156
Hutchinson, Thomas, 99
Hyam, Ronald, 120

The Iliad, 21
Impressment of American seaman, 93,
    101–3, 138
India, 90, 92, 100; Johore State, 117;
    Mahratta Confederation, 103; Mu-
    tiny of 1857, 115–16; non-violent
    resistance, 122–23
Ireland, 85–87, 89–90, 122; Rising of
    1798, 102
Irish in America, 96, 99, 105 n.31,
    133–34
Isis, 37–38
Islam, 56, 163. *See also* Religion
Israel, 151, 154
Italy, 112, 123

Jackson, Francis James "Copenhagen,"
    139
James, First Earl, Stanhope, 80

James I of England, 88
Japan, 50, 123, 125–26, 140–41, 146–47, 156, 160 n.28, 165–67
Jay, John, 101, 135–38
Jefferson, Thomas, 138
Jiang Jieshi (Chiang Kai-Shek), 166–67. See also Nationalist Chinese
Jiang Jingguo, 174
Ji mi (loose rein) policy of Tang, 10
Jin, Chinese state of, 3
John V Cantacuzene, Emperor of Byzantium, 78
John Comnenus, Emperor of Byzantium, 70
Johnson, Andrew, 141
Johnson, Lyndon B., 153, 168
Jones, John Paul, 99
Jordan, Sir John, 165
Julius II, Pope, 74
Jurchen tribe, 5, 15, 16
Justinian I, Emperor of Byzantium, 50, 54, 57–59, 65 n.10

Kaegi, Walter F., Jr., 51
Kaplan, Lawrence S., 95
Kellerman, Henry J., 149
Kennedy, John F., 152
Khitans, 11–15
Kissinger, Henry, 169–70
Kluge, John, 157
Kolko, Gabriel, 147
Korea, 12, 14, 153
Korean War, 148, 150, 161 n.44, 167–68

Lake, General Gerard, Viscount, 103
Latin America, relations with United States of America, 146, 156
Lattimore, Owen, 5, 49
League of Cambrai, 74
League of Venice, 70, 74
Leggett, Robert, 153
Lendrum, John, 93

Leo, Emperor of Byzantium, 49–50
Li, consort of Han Emperor Xiaowu, 4
Libya, 127
Lincoln, Abraham, 141
Liu, Jing, Han dynasty counselor, 6
Liudprand, 60
Lloyd George, David, 121, 128
Louis, King of Hungary, 72
Louis IX of France, 87
Louis XIV of France, 89
Louisiana Purchase, 138
Luan, Baoqun, 9
Lugar, Richard, 156

Macartney, Sir George, 93
Macedonia, 27, 33
Machiavelli, Niccolò, 67, 77–79, 81
Madison, James, 138–39
Mahoney, Rosemary, 173
Malcolm, Sir John, 115
Manchus, 16–17, 163
Mantua, 75
Manuel I Comnenus, Emperor of Byzantium, 55–57, 60–64, 70
Manuel II (Paleologus), Emperor of Byzantium, 57
Mao Zedong, 166
Marathon, Battle of, 24
Mardonius, 24–25
Marital alliances: Chinese, 6, 8, 11, 13, 164; Persian, 25, 53, 56–57, 62, 64, 66 n.24, 69. See also Alliances; Sex scandals; Women
Mark Antony, 40
Marshall, George Catlett, 149–50
Marshall Plan, 150
Maximis praemiis. See Bribery
McCarthy, Joseph, 149, 167
McKinley, William, 142
Medici, 77–78, 81
Memoirs (Phillipe de Commines), 73
Mercenaries, 53, 72, 74, 78, 87, 96–97
Merchants. See Trade as policy

Metternich, Clemens Lother Wenzel, Fürst von, 109
Mexico, 139–40
Meyer, John, 154
Miami, 156–57
Michael IV, the Paphlagonian, Emperor of Byzantium, 54
Michael VIII, Paleologus, Emperor of Byzantium, 56, 71
Michiel, Vitale II, Doge, 70
Milan, 73
Miletus, 23, 28
Military policy: of Britain, 87, 94, 98, 111–14, 116, 121, 123, 127; of Byzantium, 49–51, 54–55, 57; of China, 1, 5, 7, 9, 11–13, 16, 164, 168; of Japan, 166–67; of Persia, 24, 30; of Rome, 35, 37–38, 42, 44–45, 46 n.27; of United States of America, 126, 139, 149, 152, 155; of Venice, 71, 73–76. See also Mercenaries; Nuclear bomb; War
Militia, 77–78, 134
Mill, James, 92, 100
Ming dynasty, 15–17, 171
Mir Kasim, Nawab of Bengal, 92
Missionaries, 115, 129 n.21, 164. See also Religion
Mithridates. See Religion
Money, 55, 58, 81, 87, 89, 93, 107, 167. See also Gold; Wealth
Mongolia, 174
Mongols, 1, 5, 14–16, 57
Moon, Penderel, 100
Moon, Reverend Sun Myung, 153
More, Thomas, 87–88
Mosely, D. J., 31
Mughals, 90–92
Muhammad, Turkish Sultan, 57
Muhyi al-Din, Emir of Ankara, 64
Murphey, Rhoads, 91
Music, 6, 9, 14, 38, 60, 156
Mykale, Battle of, 25

Nan Tang empire, 12
Nanzhao state, 11
Naples, 73–74, 112
Nasser, Gamal Abdel, 151
Nationalist Chinese, 150–51, 166, 168, 173, 177 n.8; relations with United States of America, 166, 175
NATO, 149
Nehru, Jawaharlal, Indian Prime Minister, 151
Nero, Roman Emperor, 38
Neutrality, 74–75, 77, 81, 122
Nguyen Van Thieu, 168
Nixon, Richard M., 153, 168–69
Normans. See Anglo-Normans
Northern Han, 12
Northern Rhodesia, 120
Nuclear bomb, 124, 126, 130 n.27, 147, 153–54, 158
Nuclear Test Ban Treaty, 149

Odo of Deuil, 60–61, 63
Odyssey, 21
On the Manner of Negotiating with Princes, 19 n.37, 108
Organization for Economic Cooperation and Development, 155
Ostrogoths, 50, 54
Oswald, Richard, 98, 135
Ottoman Turks, 57, 68, 93, 118, 143. See also Turks

Padover, Saul K., 80
Padua, 68
Papal State, 70, 72–73, 77, 81
Paris, 128, 134
Park, Tongsun, 153
Parker, R.A.C., 123
Pausanias, the Spartan, 25
Peace, 52, 110, 118–19, 122, 135–36, 147, 168. See also Treaty
Peace Corps, 152
Peace of Antalcidas, 31

Peace of Callias, 27
Pechenegs, 52
People's Republic of China, 127, 157–58, 168, 171, 174, 178 n.21; border disputes, 165, 173; human rights, 172; Korean War, 161 n.44; relations with Union of Soviet Socialist Republics, 165, 169; relations with United States of America, 143, 169–70, 172, 175, 178 n.21
Pericles, 28
Persia, 26–28; relations with Athens and Sparta, 23, 25, 29, 31
Peter III of Aragon, 56
Peter the Venerable, 55
Philip III of Spain, 88
Philip of Macedon, 32
Philippine Commission, 144–45
Philippines, 41
Pierce, Franklin, 140
Piracy, 69, 75, 77, 138
Pisa, 70
Pitkin, Timothy, 93
Pitt, William, 100–101
Plague, 50, 72, 76
Platt, D.C.M., 118
Pleasure principles: for Americans, 97, 143–44, 157; for Anglo-Normans, 86, 95; for British, 121, 135; for Byzantines, 49, 64; for Chinese, 150–51; for French, 133–34; for Greeks, 22; for Romans, 35, 41; for Venetians, 67, 69, 75, 79
Plutarch, 28
Polk, James K., 141
Polo, 10
Polybius, 38
Potidaea, 24
Pragmatic Sanction, 50
Preston, William, Jr., 154
Price, Dr. Richard, 134
The Prince, 67, 77
Proclamation of 1763, 94

Profumo, John, 127, 152
Prussia, 110–11
Puritan Commonwealth, 88

Qhimin Khan, 9
Qin dynasty, 5
Qing dynasty, 17, 163–65
Quebec Act of 1774, 94
Quinn, David Beers, 86–87

Ranavoland, Queen of the Hova, 113
Rayburn, Sam, 152
Reagan, Ronald, 154, 174
Religion, 37, 41; Christianity, 38, 45, 51, 53–54, 60, 92, 102, 115, 139, 164–65; Islam, 56, 163; Roman empire, 37. See also Crusade
Rhodes, Cecil John, 120
Rhodes Fellowships, 120
Richelieu, Armand du Plessis, Duc de, 80
Roger II, Norman King, 70
Roman empire, 35–36, 43, 45 n.4, 65 n.10; in Britain, 44; Jewish Rebellion, 42
Romanus III Argyros, 54
Roosevelt, Elliott, 154
Roosevelt, Franklin D., 125–26, 146, 148, 166–67
Roosevelt, Theodore, 122, 144, 160 n.28
Root, Elihu, 145
Russia, 53, 77, 90, 93, 110, 114, 119, 142, 147. See also Union of Soviet Socialist Republics
Ryuku Islands, 9

Said, Seyyid, Sultan of Muscat and Zanziar, 113
Salamis, Battle of, 24
Salisbury, Robert Arthur Talbot Gascoyne Cecil, Marquess of, 119
Samarkand, golden peaches of, 10

Samoa, 143

Samuel, Tsar of Bulgaria, 54

Santa Anna, Antonio Lopez de, 139

Sarmiento de Acuna, Diego, Count of
Gondomar, 88

Schroeder, Paul, 116–17

Schultz, George, 171

Scots: emigration to Ireland, 87; emigration to United States of America,
95, 99; relations with Britain, 90

Scott, Peter Dale, 152, 154

Scribani, Carlo, 80

Serbia, 52, 56, 70

Seven Years War, 93, 114

Seward, William Henry, 141–42, 159
n.16

Sex scandals, 127, 152–54. See also
Marital alliance; Women

Seymour, Sir George Hamilton, 114

Shelburne, William Petty, Earl of, 135

Sherry, Michael S., 150

Shu, Chinese kingdom of, 8

Sicilian Vespers, 56

Sicily, 56, 59, 62

Silk, 4, 6–7, 9, 13–14, 172

Sima Qian, Han historian, 5

Singapore, 116–17, 123

"Six Strategies," 2

Slavery, 59, 111–12, 135–37, 141

Slevin, Peter, 156

Song, Chinese state of, 3

Song, Qi, adviser to Song Taicong, 12

Song, Zhencong, Emperor, 12

Song dynasty, 12–15, 18 n.25

Song Taicong, Emperor, 12

Soong, T. V., 166–67. See also Nationalist Chinese

Spain, 74–75, 81, 111–12, 135, 144

Sparta, 24–25, 27, 30–31

Spectacle: American, 145; Byzantine,
59–61, 63; Chinese, 9, 169–70

Spies. See Diplomacy

Spring-Rice, Sir Cecil, 122

Stamp Act, 94–95, 105 n.26

Starr, Chester, 45

Stephenson, J. E., 120

Sternsdorf, Speck von, 146

Stockwell, John, 153

Suez Canal, 119, 151

Sugar, 87, 90

Sugar Act of 1764, 94–95

Sui dynasty, 8

Sun Tzu's Art of War: The Modern
Chinese Interpretation, 17 n.7

Su Song, 14

Symeon, Archbishop of Bulgaria, 51–
52

Tacitus, 43–44

Taft, William Howard, 144–45, 160
n.28

Taiwan, 167–68, 170, 174–75. See
also Nationalist Chinese

Talleyrand-Périgord, Charles Maurice
de, Prince de Bénévent, 80, 110,
138, 158 n.9

Tang dynasty, 10–11

Tansill, Charles C., 144

Taxation, 27, 47 n.29, 53, 58, 62, 78,
91, 93–94, 108, 143–44, 155

Tea, 10, 95, 164–66, 172

Ten Books on Politics, 80

Thargelia, 28–29

Thasos, 26–27

Thatcher, Melvin P., 4

Thessalonica, 52–53, 64

Thieu, Nguyen Van, President of South
Vietnam, 168

Thirty Years War, 76

Thompson, James Westfall, 80

Thompson, Suzi (Sook Nai Park), 153

Thrace, 26, 50

Thucydides, 26, 28

Thurheim, Countess Ludovica, 109

Tibet, 10, 165, 168, 173

Townshend Act, 94, 105 n.26

Toynbee, Arnold, 54, 65 n.10
Trade as policy: for Americans, 133–
  34, 136–37, 141, 146, 148–49, 151–
  52, 157; for British, 89–91, 101,
  112, 122, 125–26; for Byzantines,
  52, 58, 62, 71; for Chinese, 4–5, 13,
  16, 164–67, 174–75; for Romans,
  39, 44; for Venetians, 55, 68–70, 72
Trajan, Emperor, 43
Treaty, 13, 68–70, 72–74, 107, 138,
  165. See also Alliances; Peace
Treaty of Bura, 165
Treaty of Chaumont, 107
Treaty of Dover, 89
Treaty of Hanover, 81
Treaty of Kiakhta, 165
Treaty of Lodi, 73
Treaty of Miletus, 29
Treaty of Nerchinsk, 165
Treaty of Paris, 108, 137
Treaty of Pavia, 69
Treaty of Shan-Yuan, 13
Treaty of Turin, 72
Tripoli, 138
Trist, Nicholas, 140
Trojan War, 21, 41
Truman, Harry, 148, 150
Tunis, 77, 138
Turfan, 10
Turks, 9–10, 54–55, 72–76; relations
  with Tang dynasty, 11. See also Ar-
  abs; Ottoman Turks

UNESCO, 148–49, 154
Union of Soviet Socialist Republics,
  124, 155, 168, 170, 172, 174; col-
  lapse of, 154; Korean War, 161 n.44;
  in Manchuria, 165; relations with
  China, 165, 169, 172; relations with
  United States of America, 151, 170.
  See also Russia
United Nations, 148, 152, 154, 174
United States of America: colonization,

137, 143, 145; cultural exchanges,
  148–49, 151; Department of State,
  156, 158; economic assistance, 146,
  148, 150, 152, 154–56; military,
  149; relations with China, 172; relations with Cuba, 144; relations with
  Japan, 125–26, 140, 167; relations
  with Russia, 154–55, 170. See also
  American Revolution; Civil War;
  French and Indian War
Uros II Milutin, Serbian King, 57
U.S.–China People's Friendship Association, 172
Utopia, 87–88
Uzbeks, 14

Vandals, 43, 49
Van Gulik, Robert, 1
Venice, 55–56, 58–59, 61, 67–72, 110;
  conquered, 68; cost of diplomacy,
  73; cost of warfare, 76; influence on
  Renaissance, 81 n.1
Vercengetorix, 40
Vergil, 41
Vestal Virgins, 37
Vienna, 108, 111–12. See also Con-
  gress of Vienna
Vietnam, 12, 153, 168, 173, 178 n.23
Villiers, Barbara, Lady Castelmaine, 89
Vladimir, Prince of Russia, 53, 60
von Stoeckl, Edouard, 142

Wales, 85–86
Wall building, 16–17, 19 n.44, 50, 91
Wang Gungwu, 10
Wang Zhaojun, 8
War: for Britain, 92, 96, 103, 114,
  117–18, 135; for Germany, 122; for
  Italians, 73; for Japan, 125–26, 148;
  for Mexico, 140; for Spain, 144; for
  the Turks, 75–76. See also Military
  policy; Neutrality; Nuclear Bomb

Warfare, 91; aerial, 124; naval, 68, 121, 123

War for American Independence. *See* American Revolution

War of 1812, 102

War of Chioggia, 72

Warren, Mercy, 93

Washington, George, 101, 136–37

Wealth, 67, 79, 85, 119, 164. *See also* Gold; Money

Webster, Daniel, 112–13

Webster-Ashburton Treaty, 112

Wellesley, Governor General Arthur, Duke of Wellington, 103, 105 n.23

Western Zhou, 2

Whiskey Rebellion, 137

Whitworth, Charles, 111

Wilhelm II, Kaiser, 145

Wilson, Charles, 151

Wilson, Woodrow, 122

Women: African, 120; American, 97, 99, 134, 149; British attitudes, 114–18, 120, 129 n.22; Burmese, 117; Byzantine, 58; Chinese, 1–4, 18 n.14, 164, 173; at Congress of Vienna, 108–11; French, 108; German, 147, 149; Greek, 28; and Hessian deserters, 96–97, 99; Hong Kong, 173; Irish, 86–87, 89, 102–3; Italian, 146; Japanese, 140–41, 148; Korean, 153; Malaysian, 117; Persian, 10, 25, 29; Philippine, 45; Roman, 37, 40; Tibetan, 176 n.3; Venetian, 75. *See also* Marital alliances; Sex scandals

Xenia, 22

Xenophon, 26, 30

Xerxes, 24–25

Xiaowu, Han Emperor, 4

Xiongnu, 5–8, 18 n.14

Xi Shi, 3, 13–14

Yang, Emperor, 9

Yangdi, Emperor, 8–9

Yang Giuan, 8

You, Emperor, 2

Yue, Chinese state of, 3

Zhang Qi, adviser to Song Taicong, 12

Zhang Qian, 7, 11

Zheng, Chinese state of, 3

Zhou Enlai, Chinese Premier, 169–70

Zoe, Empress, 52

About the Author

THOMAS A. BRESLIN is Vice President for Research and Associate Professor of International Relations at Florida International University. Professor Breslin has published three earlier books and numerous articles in scholarly journals.

www.ingramcontent.com/pod-product-compliance
Lightning Source LLC
Chambersburg PA
CBHW062026270326
41929CB00014B/2329